Assessment and therapy for young dysfluent children: family interaction

To Michael Palin
For his generosity and support in helping to establish the Michael Palin Centre for Stammering Children and their Families.

Assessment and therapy for young dysfluent children: family interaction

Lena Rustin, Willie Botterill, Elaine Kelman

W

Whurr Publishers Ltd
London

First published 1996 by
Whurr Publishers Ltd
19b Compton Terrace, London N1 2UN, England

British Library Cataloguing in Publication Data
A catalogue record for this book is available from the British Library.

ISBN 1-897635-55-9

Contents

Acknowledgements

We would like to express our grateful thanks to Jane Fry for her contribution to the text. We would also like to thank our colleagues, Rob Spence, Frances Cook and Diana de Grunwald, for their help and encouragement during the preparation of this book. We are most grateful to Francilla Morris for typing the many drafts of the manuscript.

Note to readers

Pronouns *she* and *he* are used to refer to therapist and client respectively, generally reflecting professional preponderances.

Foreword

Some approach childhood stuttering in a 'full-theory-ahead-and-damn-the-data' manner. Conversely, others approach children who stutter in a 'use-it-if-it-works-and-don't-ask-why' fashion. In this book, Lena Rustin, Willie Botterill and Elaine Kelman do neither. Instead, writing the thin line between these two extremes, the three authors show that we can make further progress in the treatment of childhood stuttering if we ground our empirically derived clinical method in relevant theory and provide factual motivation for that which we do clinically. The authors do this by combining their years of clinical experience together with modern-day research and theory to provide a cohesive, motivated approach to the management of childhood stuttering. Many laudatory words can be used to describe this clinically salient book, but perhaps three capture its essence: interaction, flexibility and continuity.

Rustin, Botterill and Kelman make clear the importance of *interaction* between the child and his environment when trying to assess and treat children who stutter. Consistently recognising the bidirectionality of this interaction these three authors, from the first chapter to the last, weave a sturdy net of ideas and approaches that attempts to capture salient aspects of the child, his environment and interactions between the two. Approaching this interaction from four different, but interrelated perspectives — speech production, language/linguistics, psychoemotional and sociocultural — the authors establish, by means of their assessment procedures, a foundation of understanding of each child upon which they raise a treatment superstructure that is adapted to the elements of each child.

Given the capturing powers of their observational net, the authors' approach is quite *flexible* in that once they establish the child's concerns through their assessment, they are able to attend to the special needs of the child and the child's family whilst being able to deal with that which is common between this child and all others. Such flexibility also comes from the fact that few relevant considerations appear to be overlooked and the fact that the authors provide a rationale for assessing the many subtle but significant variables that may affect the child's speech fluency, e.g. disturbances to the equilibrium of the family due to problems of a sibling.

Making explicit one of the more thorough diagnostic approaches to be found in the entire literature pertaining to childhood stuttering, the authors provide a *continuity* of approach that ties together the whole of their clinical practice. For example, from the very beginning, by insisting that both parents come to the first assessment appointments, through to the end, whereby both parents are involved in the maintenance phase these authors' attempt to ground treatment in assessment, much as their attempt to ground practice in theory, leads to a continuity of thought and practice that serves to make their approach logical as well as defendable, to both consumers and professionals alike.

Written throughout in a straightforward manner, the practising clinician should find it easy to grasp their approach and ideas. Liberally supported throughout with clinical observations and case studies, the book seldom strays from its central topic — assessment and treatment of childhood stuttering — and this focus should provide a strong incentive to anyone interested in learning more about the assessment and treatment of childhood stuttering.

Reading this book often reminds one of looking through an observation window at master clinicians plying their trade. In this case, though, we not only read about the art and science of their approach, but what these clinicians believe they are doing, when and why. Thus, although it is not possible for us to actually observe these three authors providing clinical services or interview them afterwards about same, this book gives us a somewhat similar experience. Enjoy. I think you will!

Edward G Conture
Syracuse University
USA

Chapter 1
Introduction

This book aims to provide a comprehensive but essentially practical approach to the treatment of early childhood dysfluency. The complexity, diversity and variability of this heterogeneous disorder is a challenging prospect for clinicians. For many years theorists such as Wendell Johnson (1959) advocated that parents should ignore the problem. Furthermore, remission rates of up to 80% were cited in the research (Andrew and Harris, 1964; Bloodstein, 1987). It therefore became common practice to counsel parents of dysfluent children under the age of 7 that they would probably grow out of it.

However, it is clear that dysfluency emerges in its simplest form at the time of onset, before it has become compounded by environmental, developmental and psycho-social influences. There is also increasing evidence from recent research indicating that early intervention with dysfluent children is highly effective (Starkweather and Gottwald, 1990; Meyers and Woodford, 1992). Thus the earlier we can identify the features that put a child at risk of long-term dysfluency and develop procedures that will provide the best opportunity for their resolution, the more likely we are to be able to prevent the development of a chronic stuttering problem.

Onset and development of stuttering

Most stuttering begins in early childhood. It usually appears from 18 months to 12 years but is most commonly reported between 2–5 years at a time of phenomenal physical, linguistic, neurological and cognitive growth. Recent research seems to suggest that the onset of stuttering is rather earlier than previously reported. Yairi and Ambrose (1992) indicate a clear tendency for its occurrence under 3 years of age, and found evidence that girls begin stuttering significantly earlier than boys. This gender difference is reflected in the commensurately earlier age at which a girl's developing central nervous system matures and seems to support the evidence for a close relationship between the onset of stuttering and the development of speech and language skills.

Although in the past there has been much discussion in the literature about the commonplace circumstances, the lack of identifiably provocative events, and typically gradual appearance of early stuttering (Johnson, 1959; Van Riper, 1973), evidence is beginning to emerge to the contrary. Van Riper (1971) and Yairi (1983, 1992) conclude that in many cases the onset of stuttering is clear, well defined, and relatively brief. Yairi also noted that severe stuttering had a strong tendency to be linked with a sudden onset. Further significant data was reported by Yairi and Ambrose (1992) in a longitudual study of stuttering in children relating to the marked deceleration over time in the mean frequency of 'stuttering-like' dysfluencies. These authors report that much of this reduction took place near the end of the first year post-onset, indicating group differences between chronic and recovering stutterers which became distinct by approximately 20 months post-onset. This evidence clearly indicates the importance of obtaining accurate information about the timing and circumstances pertaining to the onset of dysfluency as it facilitates the identification of those children who are likely to need early intervention in order to avoid the development of a chronic problem.

Remission

It is difficult to be definitive about the proportion of children who will recover without therapy as the research reports wide variations. Andrews et al. (1983) reported recovery rates from 23% to 80% when they reviewed research from all available studies. With evidence that as many as 80% of children might recover without help it is easy to understand why so many professionals advised parents that they should not worry about it and the problem would 'go away'. It is our view, however, that this is no longer acceptable. Starkweather (1987) states that 20%, and perhaps as many as 50%, of children whose parents notice excessively repetitive speech behaviour will go on to exhibit chronic dysfluency. Although the reported figures are so variable, the body of evidence that we have available indicates that an in-depth understanding of all the factors that contribute to the development of early childhood dysfluency is essential in order to be able to make an informed statement about whether a particular child is at risk of developing a stutter.

Normal dysfluency or early stuttering?

Whether stuttering emerges from normal non-fluency or is qualitatively different from the beginning continues to cause controversy and no discussion of early stuttering is complete without reference to this debate. Indeed, there is evidence for both arguments. Normal dysfluencies are generally accepted to be revisions, interjections, repetitions, prolongations and pauses. Up to 10% of a child's speech between 2–3½ years may contain such dysfluencies and for some this percentage may be even higher (Yairi, 1981; Wexler and Mysak, 1982; DeJoy and Gregory, 1985).

Riley (1984) suggests a number of predictors which include phonatory arrest and articulatory posturing as possible indications of chronic dysfluency. Van Riper (1982) suggests that any signs of tension, rise in pitch, increasing length of prolongations or blocks are highly significant. Van Riper (1982) and Gregory and Hill (1984) suggest that disruption of the phonation between repetitions or the emergence of the 'schwa' vowel are also predictive. Since then studies by Howell and Vause (1986), Howell and Williams (1992), and Yaruss and Conture (1993) have cast doubts on the role of the 'schwa' vowel. They do suggest, however, that there is a change in the part-word repetitions of children who stutter (shorter, less intense, but *not* 'schwa' vowels) and that the duration of the transition from the consonant to the vowel may provide clues about the chronicity of the dysfluency. As well as qualitative changes, there is also evidence that early stuttering features a higher frequency of dysfluencies, with more than 10% being considered significant (Yairi, 1983; Gregory and Hill, 1984; Yairi and Lewis, 1984). Conture and Caruso (1987) consider a child to be at risk where three or more within-word dysfluencies occur per 100 words. Research has also suggested that repetitions that exceed two units are a cause for concern, especially if the rhythm is also disrupted (Yairi, 1983; Gregory and Hill, 1984; Yairi and Lewis, 1984).

Finally, however, Yairi et al. presented a paper at the ASHA Convention 1994, which suggests that the severity of the symptom (qualitative or quantitative) is not a reliable indicator of chronicity. The preliminary results of this longitudinal study seem to suggest that other factors, such as co-occurring speech and language difficulties, may be more reliable predictors.

Peters and Guitar (1991) refer to 'borderline' stutterers as being subtly different from normally dysfluent children but also feel that there are no single behaviours that distinguish one group from the other.

Variability

One of the confounding factors associated with early childhood dysfluency is its variability. We have frequently been frustrated in our attempts to make an accurate assessment of a child's dysfluency as, much to the consternation of their parents, children may become unusually fluent on the assessment occasion. We have therefore found it imperative to listen to the descriptions given by parents who are extremely concerned, frequently with justification. They may also be able to provide a tape recording made at home for further analysis. In such cases, as with all others, a full assessment of both parents and child should be undertaken and not until all factors have been considered should any decisions be taken regarding diagnosis, prognosis or therapy.

A theoretical framework

The procedures described in this book are an attempt to look at all of the above issues and to provide a practical approach to the young dysfluent population that takes into account the needs of the individual child, the parents, and the environment within which they function.

The guiding principles of the approach that we have developed are that any coherent therapy procedures must have their roots firmly established in a sound theoretical framework. This framework should be wide enough to subsume within it the range of possibilities presented in clinic. It should furnish clinicians with a rationale and an explanation for each case and direct them to the intervention procedures necessary for remediation. This should also be presented to parents in a format that is easily understood. Sharing information from the beginning establishes a relationship whereby the value of parents is recognised and undisputed, the child is seen in the context of the family and the parents are seen as the experts on their child. Our theoretical framework draws on the work of many authors and provides a brief overview of current thinking about the ways in which we can increase our understanding of the young dysfluent child. The idea that stuttering is a heterogeneous disorder is not new. Conture (1982) and Conture and Caruso (1987) describe stuttering as a complex interaction between the child's environment and the skills and abilities the child brings to that environment. Cooper (1987) based his therapeutic approach on the assumption that stuttering 'is the result of multiple coexisting physiological and psychological factors'.

An interactionist model of the development of early dysfluency and stuttering is further described by Gregory and Hill (1984), Wall and Myers (1984), Rustin (1987) and Starkweather (1987). The underlying assumption to this interactionist model suggests that there is a neurophysiological predisposition to the problem with a variety of developmental, linguistic and psychosocial factors playing an important role in the emergence of the disorder. We share this multifactorial approach to the development of dysfluency and, in addition, draw attention to the complex and bidirectional interaction of these factors. In describing the framework which we have adopted, we have divided the factors into four subgroups to try to conceptualize the problem systematically. The divisions we have made are somewhat arbitrary as in reality no such divisions can be made. These are:

- Physiological factors.
- Linguistic factors.
- Sociocultural or environmental factors.
- Psychological/emotional factors.

Dividing the factors in this way helps to focus the research and discussion in the literature and provides a framework for understanding each child's particular pattern of vulnerabilities and, finally, helps us to formulate a therapy package designed to ameliorate these conditions.

Physiological factors

Role of genetics

There is undoubted evidence of an inherited predisposition towards stuttering (Pauls, 1990). Bloodstein (1987), in a review of 13 family studies, found that more people who stutter reported a family history of stuttering than fluent speakers. Andrews et al. (1983) estimated that the incidence of stuttering among first-degree relatives of people who stutter is more than three times that in the general population. The research also demonstrates that males are more likely to stutter than females, but that first-degree relatives of females who stutter are at greatest risk (Kidd, 1977; Kidd, Kidd and Records, 1978). Twin studies support a genetic factor by finding a higher concordance in monozygotic twins than in dizygotic twins (Howie, 1981; Martin 1990). However, the picture is complicated by the fact that researchers also provide compelling evidence for the influence of environmental factors interacting with genetics (Cox, Seider and Kidd, 1984) demonstrated in particular by the discordance for stuttering in identical twins reared apart (Farber, 1981). In conclusion, it seems that some, as yet unknown, factors appear to be inherited but that other variables may need to be present in order to trigger this predisposition.

Hemispheric processing

There is also a growing body of evidence to support the idea that there are differences in the central nervous system (CNS) functioning of people who stutter. In particular, differences have been reported in hemispheric processing. Moore and Boberg (1987), in reviewing the research, state that 'stutterers do not typically use left hemispheric strategies to process language as do normal speakers' and that there is some evidence demonstrating a shift from right to left hemispheric processing following successful therapy (Boberg et al., 1983; Moore, 1984). Peters and Guitar (1991) discuss a possible link between this apparent increase in right hemispheric activity which is usually associated with emotional expression and stuttering, and conclude that 'fluency may be especially vulnerable to emotional disruption then because of "cross-talk" between speech and emotional expression'.

Reaction times

Further evidence of a neuro-physiological predisposition to stutter comes from the considerable research which has been conducted into the reaction times of people who stutter. Some of this research has shown that, as a group, adults who stutter have slower reaction times across a variety of activities, e.g. vocal reaction times, respiration and articulation (Adler and Starkweather, 1979; Peters and Hulstijn, 1987). Interestingly, research has also found that children who stutter show similarly delayed reaction times (Cullinan and Springer, 1980; Till, Reich, Dickey and Sieber, 1983). However, as with many areas of research in this field, there are many individual differences and, as Bloodstein (1987; 1995) pointed out, the differences between people who stutter and fluent speakers have shown themselves to be neither necessary nor sufficient to create stuttering.*

Acoustic studies

These studies have looked at the speed and coordination of speech movements during fluent speech of stutterers and found that they tend to have slower consonant–vowel transitions and speech movements generally (Starkweather and Myers, 1979; Zimmerman, 1980a). There is considerable debate as to the reasons for these findings, e.g. delay in processing signals, a slower mechanism working at its normal rate or increased tension as a reaction to stuttered speech (Starkweather, 1987). More recently there has been some concern as to whether these 'fluent' tokens contain 'subperceptual' instances of stuttering (Armson and Kalinowski, 1994; Lees, 1994). These studies undoubtedly provide further evidence for a neuro-physiological predisposition to stutter.

In conclusion, it seems that some people who stutter have disturbances in cerebral laterality, laryngeal motor control or in their processing of signals. These can occur singly or in combination, but it is most likely that it is the interaction of these features with other linguistic, environmental or psychological features that will provide the conditions necessary for stuttering to develop.

*For further reading on reaction times, see Adams, Freeman and Conture (1985).

Linguistic factors

The onset of stuttering is most commonly recorded between the ages of 2–5 years and coincides with intensive physical growth and neurological maturation. These physical changes are competing with a rapid expansion in cognitive and linguistic development for the available neurological resources. The relationship between the demands being placed on these systems and fluency is complex and not clear; however, there is some agreement amongst theorists that where the demand being placed on these resources outstrips the child's capacity to process and organise them, dysfluency will result (Starkweather, 1987; 1990). Dalton and Hardcastle (1977) discuss the relationship between speech and language development and fluency and state 'the ever increasing demands on linguistic competence and articulatory proficiency is a major factor in the onset of some dysfluency', whereas Andrews et al. (1983) conclude that dysfluency is most likely to occur 'at a time when an explosive growth in language ability outstrips a still immature speech motor apparatus'. Research in the field suggests a reciprocal relationship between early speech and language development and dysfluency. There is evidence that children who stutter tend to be later in saying their first words and phrases and later acquiring intelligible speech (Accordi et al., 1983). They also perform poorly on tests of linguistic ability at an early age (Bloodstein, 1987; 1995) and demonstrate an increase in dysfluencies as language becomes more complex (Bernstein-Ratner and Sih, 1987). More recent research seems to indicate that the length of utterance may be as important as the complexity in determining whether an utterance is stuttered or not (Gaines, Runyan and Meyers, 1991; Weiss and Zebrowski, 1992; Logan and Conture, 1995). There are also studies indicating that dysfluencies occur more frequently at clause boundaries where language is being formulated (Wall, 1977; Wall, Starkweather and Cairns, 1981).

Finally, dysfluent children tend to have more articulatory problems (Conture, 1990) lending weight to the theory that these individuals' speech motor control systems are vulnerable. Clearly, children who stutter are less skilled verbally (Wall, 1977; Kline and Starkweather, 1979) and often have an identifiable speech and language delay. These identified factors that are related to speech and language development are not enough to cause the dysfluency but clearly where they are present, they increase the likelihood of fluency breakdown. It is interesting to note the results of a study by Merits-Patterson and Reed (1981) which shows that children with delayed language development sometimes begin to stutter when they encounter the more demanding environment of the language clinic. In these cases it appears that the language disorder in itself was not enough to trigger the dysfluency, but the increased pressure on the child to perform as a result of language therapy was.

Environmental/sociocultural factors

The role of environmental factors has been widely acknowledged by virtually all the contributors to our understanding of the nature of stuttering. Glasner (1970) and Sheehan (1975) emphasised the child's interpersonal relationships in the family as primary in the development of the problem. There are others, including those who have investigated the genetics of stuttering (Kidd, 1983) who believe that environmental factors interact with physiological predispositions (Van Riper, 1982; Riley and Riley, 1983; Gregory, 1985, 1986).

These environmental factors include all the many communicative and interpersonal stimuli that young children experience. As the major source of these experiences comes from within the family, the attitudes, child-rearing practices, and interrelationships of family members are profoundly relevant. The research in this area is often conflicting, however, Bloodstein's (1987; 1995) review of these studies suggests that a sizeable proportion of the parents of children who stutter appear to be, in varying degrees, 'demanding', 'over anxious' or 'perfectionist' in their child-rearing practices. Competitive pressure for achievement or conformity has been established as a contributing factor to stuttering behaviour. Prins (1983) contributed further to this view by describing more general sources of environmental stress and uncertainty in the household that contribute to the child's difficulties, such as:

- Erratic planning and conduct of routine daily activities, e.g. mealtimes, bedtimes.
- Unsettling time pressures.
- Unpredictable changes in the family constellation, e.g. lodgers, grandparents, parental absences.
- Behavioural demands the child is unable to meet.
- Insufficient time attending to a child's individual needs.

It is clear that these stresses alone do not produce stuttering but may be able to trigger the behaviour in a child who is constitutionally so predisposed. Added to these more general pressures within the family are those that relate specifically to the communicative environment, and the demands being placed on a child's developing speech and language system by significant people in or around the family. As the child's capacity for language and fluency increases so will the expectations of those with whom he is communicating. When the child's speech and language systems are unable to meet the communicative demands placed upon it, stuttering will result (Starkweather, 1987). Meyers and Freeman (1985a, 1985b, 1985c) demonstrated that adults tend to talk more rapidly when talking to children who stutter and to interrupt them more often, providing evidence that the child's stuttering influences the mother's rate in a reciprocal and bidirectional manner. Starkweather and Gottwald (1984) found it was possible to predict the extent of a child's recovery by the parent's ability to reduce their speech rate. Newman and Smit (1989) demonstrated that the speech production of a child (rate, interruptions and fluency) was influenced by an adult who varied the length of response time. Where the adult increased latency the child responded with a similar increase in latency and also became more fluent.

The communicative environment can also be responsible for making demands on a child's ability to formulate language (Wall and Myers, 1984; Starkweather and Gottwald, 1990). Parents using long, less frequently occurring words, as well as longer syntactically and semantically complex sentences, may provide models that the child tries to emulate and as the child attempts more complex linguistic structures so the amount of dysfluency increases (Crystal, 1987).

Frequent questions, demands for speech performance, and negative reactions to dysfluency also place children under extra pressure to perform in an acceptable manner, and have been described by many authors as contributing to environmental stressors that can affect the development of dysfluency. Peters and Guitar (1991) reviewing the stresses noted by several clinicians as being likely to increase stuttering, state as follows:

- Stressful adult models
    - Rapid speech rate
    - Complex syntax
    - Polysyllabic vocabulary
    - Use of more than one language in the home
- Stressful speaking situations for the child
    - Competition for speaking
    - Hurried when speaking
    - Frequent interruptions
    - Frequent questions
    - Demand for display speech
    - Excited when speaking
    - Loss of listener attention
    - Many things to say

It is clear that environmental factors have a role to play in the early development and ultimately in the remediation of early childhood dysfluency, since these factors are particularly amenable to change. However, it is important to remember that these factors are not in themselves sufficient or necessary to cause stuttering.

Psychological and emotional factors

When parents and children are stressed or anxious it affects the way they think, behave and communicate. The child's actions are to a degree, governed by characteristics of the family's system, and may be responding to stresses within the family unit or be contributing to stressing other members within the family system (Minuchin, 1974).

The stuttering child lives within a family and is a member of a social system within which he learns to adapt. It is essential therefore to understand the individual functioning of the parents and the child, but also to consider the marital dyad within the family. It is also helpful to explore the personalities involved and the strategies they employ for managing emotional issues, stress or changes in life events. Reviews of the research into the personality and adjustment of stutterers find no convincing evidence that they are different from fluent individuals (Bloch and Goodstein, 1971; Van Riper, 1982; Bloodstein, 1993). However, there is some evidence that stutterers are often regarded by their parents as being 'nervous', and exhibiting more fears, nightmares, enuresis, fighting, etc. This is a view supported by Rustin and Purser (1991) who found in addition a significant proportion of the children in their sample were described as shy, withdrawn and/or worriers. Although there is no evidence in the literature that parents of stuttering children show any distinct personality deviations (Bloodstein, 1987; 1995), there are some differences in their attitudes.

Children who are predisposed to stutter and whose speech and language functions are not yet optimally localised, may be especially vulnerable to the effect that emotions and feelings have on all motor functions, including speech. There is a complex and reciprocal relationship between these systems which Peters and Guitar (1991) suggest may permit 'cross-talk' or interference between the limbic system (structures and pathways involved in the regulation and expression of emotion) and the structures and pathways used for speech and language. Clinical evidence for this interrelationship between emotional excitement, anxiety or distress and dysfluency is readily available, and includes events such as moving home, changes in nursery or caretaker, divorce, or death of a family member (Starkweather, 1987). High levels of excitement have also been associated with an increase in dysfluencies and are often accompanied by a faster speech rate. Children are particularly susceptible to the anticipation and gathering crescendo of events, such as birthdays and Christmas, and will exhibit similar behaviours when they feel they have something of great importance to relate in a hurry. It is our clinical experience that children who are neuro-physiologically vulnerable to stuttering may be especially prone to difficulty when their emotional state interferes with their neural circuitry for speech.

We have mentioned marital discord as one of the emotional stresses for both parents and the child. The importance of the role of the parents in the conceptualisation of the child's problem is supported by research and literature in family therapy. Falloon (1988) stresses the importance of assessing the marital relationship, and states that failure to do so would be to ignore a major contributory factor to the child's problem. Furthermore, a poor marital relationship can influence treatment effectiveness since a cooperative set between parents is necessary in order to carry out essential aspects of a parent training programme. The importance of this cannot be underestimated, as an undetected marital problem may well undermine all efforts to involve the parents in a successful therapy programme. Parental discord or divorce ranks second and third in Holmes and Rahe's (1967) *Social Adjustment Rating Scale*, number one being the death of a spouse. Research by Miller (1975) and Reisinger, Frangia and Hoffman (1976) lends support to the idea that the state of the marital relationship can adversely affect the outcome of parent training programmes. In addition, Christensen et al. (1983) showed that marital discord was also related to parental perceptions of, and negative behaviour towards, the child. These findings suggest that the child may be the scapegoat for parental distress in the marriage. It has undoubtedly been our experience that the child's dysfluency can become the distracter in the family, and helping the parents address their marital difficulties can be a pivotal point in therapy.

Another equally important source of stress within families is caused by the experience of loss, and in particular death, the effect of which will depend on the extent and proximity of the loss to the family. Whilst any encounter with death will have an impact, the manner in which a family copes will provide considerable insight into the ways in which the family functions. We have found the instinct of many parents is to try to protect their children from the pain of bereavement, so that in some cases, a conspiracy develops to conceal the death. This does not allow the necessary psychological transitions to take place within the family, and creates an environment in which grief and mourning are not accepted, supported or valued. Human beings, old or young, need to mourn in response to loss and, if deprived of this experience, will suffer psychologically, physically or both. It is essential, therefore, for parents to allow themselves and their children to mourn. Kübler-Ross (1969) describes the difficulties faced by children who have been excluded from the experience of a death in the family. The child senses that something is wrong and begins to distrust adults who avoid his questions and suspicions, or provide gifts as a substitute for an unacknowledged loss. The child may go on to suffer unresolved guilt and anger without the means to cope with it. Furthermore, losses can be of two kinds:

- Physical: this may include losing a friend or an object of sentimental value.

- Symbolic: such as divorce or loss of job and status.

Both these states will initiate a process of grief within the family. Feelings of sorrow, anxiety, depression, anger and guilt are common reactions to the experience of loss. The key to successful management of these feelings is facilitating family support, by opening up flexible lines of communication between family members. Distorted, unclear and disqualifying messages are associated with family disturbance (Rando, 1984). The stresses placed on family members by the experience of loss are not to be underestimated and therefore should be explored and understood in the context of their effect on the dysfluent child.

Summary

This interactionist model underpins our philosophy and provides a rationale for our treatment. It is the complex interaction between the factors we have described that allows us to appreciate and understand the complexity and diversity of each dysfluent child. It provides the framework within which we can isolate the particular features in each child's history and environment that have contributed to the development and maintenance of the problem. Ultimately, it helps the therapist to select the relevant constituents of a treatment package uniquely designed to meet the needs of each dysfluent child and family. All the questions from the Parent Interview and Child Assessment procedures described in subsequent chapters are designed to seek further clarification of issues relevant within each of the four factors we have described here.

Chapter 2
Child Assessment

Introduction

We have described a multifactorial model for understanding the complexity and diversity of childhood dysfluency that includes physiological, linguistic, psychological and environmental factors. If we also accept the heterogeneity of this disorder then any assessment would have to include a comprehensive and searching range of procedures.

The next four chapters will describe in detail the extensive assessment procedure we have developed, based on this theoretical framework. The aim of these procedures is that parents and clinicians will ultimately share an understanding of the nature of the problem from which will emerge a therapeutic strategy, based on these findings. There are four components to the assessment:

- **The Child Assessment** provides detailed and accurate information about the current status of the child's speech and language development (linguistic factors). The child interview also provides some insight into the child's level of awareness of the problem (psychological/emotional factors).
- **The Interaction Assessment** gives detailed information about the child's communicative environment (environmental/sociocultural factors).
- **The Parent Interview** has been designed to provide further detailed information relating to the four factors. For example, the questions concerning the child's physical health, birth history and family history will indicate whether there are physiological and/or genetic factors that would make this child more vulnerable to fluency breakdown. Details of the child's speech and language development and communication skills will provide insight into possible linguistic factors. Similarly, there are questions about the child's school/nursery environment, siblings, and child-rearing practices within the family which

will reveal factors in the sociocultural environment that may be significant. Finally, there are questions that explore the emotional and psychological factors that might be relevant to the child or to the family as a whole; for example, personality traits, relationships and the experience of loss, bereavement or change.

- **The Formulation** is a summary of the assessment findings which is presented to the parents as a basis for remediation.

All the information gathered during the child assessment, the interaction assessment and the parent interview falls into one of the four factors described in Chapter 1 as the basis for our theoretical model. It may assist clinicians to see how this is achieved so Table 2.1 takes each factor in turn and demonstrates where the information is obtained in the assessment procedure. For example, evidence of sibling rivalry may be obtained from the parental interview (p.155) as well as from the Child Assessment (p.146).

The assessment is conducted over two sessions. The first session involves the parents, the child and the therapist. A video is made of each parent playing with their child (see Chapter 3 on assessment of parent–child interaction for further details). The child is then assessed while the parents observe the proceedings, which takes approximately one hour. The therapist will then make an appointment for both parents to return within one week to complete the Parent Interview. The second session involves both parents and the therapist in an interview procedure that lasts approximately 2-3 hours, at the end of which the therapist will make a summary of the findings from all the assessments and make recommendations for therapy.

Child assessment

The child assessment is a comprehensive procedure which evaluates the child's communication as a whole, rather than focusing on fluency in isolation. Particular attention is paid to the child's linguistic ability: receptive language, vocabulary, syntactic, pragmatic and word-finding ability. These are all essential skills which underpin fluency and any deficit may have implications for the remediation programme. The areas of assessment are as follows:

- General behaviour.
- Cognitive skills.
- Receptive, expressive and pragmatic language.
- Social skills.
- Dysfluency.
- Attitudes.

Table 2.1 Factors for understanding childhood dysfluency

	Parental interview (Pages)	*Child assessment* (Pages)	*Interaction assessment* (Pages)
Physiological			
family history	157, 159	146	
developmental history	153, 154, 157, 159, 161		
general health	153, 157		
neurological signs	153, 154, 157, 159, 161		
attention disorder	153, 156, 160	141	148
motor coordination	153, 154, 156, 161	141	148
motor development	153, 154, 161		
perceptual problems	153, 154, 156, 160	141	148
speech motor processes	153, 154, 161	144	148
birth history	161		
Linguistic			
receptive language	154	142, 143, 144	148
expressive language	154, 161	143, 144	148
word retrieval		143, 143, 147	148
phonology	154	143, 144	148
rate of speech		145, 147	148
bilingualism	151	142, 143, 144	148
speech and language development	154, 161	141–147	148
response to dysfluency	152, 162	145, 146, 147	148
onset of dysfluency	152	146	
nature of dysfluency	152	145, 147	148
awareness	152, 162	145, 146, 147	148
Environmental/sociocultural			
teasing	155, 156	146	
nursery/school	156	146	
parental expectations	153–162		148
linguistic environment	154, 155, 156, 160		148
communicative environment	152, 154–157	146	148
child-rearing	153, 154, 156, 158–162	146	148
management issues	152, 153, 154, 156, 159–162		148
eating routines	153		
sleeping routines	153, 159, 161		
family circumstances	156, 157, 158, 159–162	146	
sibling issues	152, 155, 156, 159, 161	146	
Psychological/emotional			
marital relationship	156, 160		
changes in care	156, 159, 160		
bereavement loss	156, 158		
separations	154, 156, 162		
personality: mother	155, 157		148
personality: father	155, 157		148
child: personality traits	154, 155, 161, 162	141, 146	148
reinforcers	152, 153, 154, 155, 161		148
parents' upbringing	158, 159		

The information is obtained by use of a variety of formal and informal tasks and measures. This is then recorded on the Child Assessment form (see Appendix I), which, when completed, provides an in-depth and comprehensive review of the child's communicative performance. The assessment procedure takes approximately one hour to administer and is structured as described below, in order to ensure that even a 2½-year-old child should be able to attend and cooperate throughout

Suggested format of child assessment

1. Cognitive task, e.g. simple formboard.
2. Assessment of comprehension using objects, pictures and commands.
3. Cognitive task, e.g. formboard.
4. *British Picture Vocabulary Scales*.
5. Cognitive tasks, e.g. wooden abacus.
6. Renfrew *Word Finding Vocabulary Scales*.
7. Goodenough *Draw-a-Man Test*.
8. Language-eliciting task using LDA *What's Wrong Pictures*.
9. Child interview.

Parents observe the assessment, preferably using a two-way mirror or remote TV unit, or seated at a distance in the assessment room. This makes parents feel an integral part of the assessment and treatment process from the onset of therapy. If parents are seated in the assessment room they are asked not to interrupt or participate in the procedure. They are also reassured that there will be ample opportunity for questions and discussion at a later stage.

We now refer to the Child Assessment Form (see appendix1).

General behaviour

GENERAL BEHAVIOUR

SEPARATION

CO-OPERATION

MANNER

ANXIETY/TENSION

ATTENTION

FIDGETING

Separation

If the child assessment is conducted with the parents observing from a viewing room we note how the child reacts to this separation. It has been our experience that it is unusual for children to be upset when parents go into the viewing room, as they are by now accustomed to the surroundings and settled by the interaction assessment. The clinician may, if necessary, continue in free play until the child is ready to cooperate with the formal assessment. However, if the child is reluctant to separate from the parents, the clinician should note the child's reactions as well as the parents' management of the situation. It could be that the parents are more anxious about the separation than the child and are perpetuating the clinging behaviour.

Cooperation

It is useful to record the child's willingness and ability to cooperate with the tasks. The structure of the assessment generally precludes uncooperative behaviour and children enjoy the material involved. However, on rare occasions, children have refused to cooperate and parents may be enlisted to engage the child in the required activities.

Manner

The child's response to both the clinician and the assessment should be recorded. Most preschool children settle quickly into a situation which has age-appropriate toys and activities, adapting rapidly to the new environment. It is important that the clinical setting should be conducive to such a response, and that the play material on display is diverting and will engage the child's interest. Similarly, the clinician's manner should facilitate the child's adjustment to the situation — adopting an appropriate balance of enthusiasm and gentleness. It is worth noting if the child presents as exceptionally withdrawn or passive, as well as if there is difficulty establishing a rapport.

Anxiety/tension

Observations are recorded of any non-verbal or verbal behaviour indicating high levels of anxiety; this may include facial expressions, repetitive body movements, rigid posture, or general unease. It should also be noted if these behaviours are specific to episodes of dysfluency or are more generally apparent.

Attention

The child's attention control is evaluated according to whether he is able to control his own attention over a period of time despite external distractions or whether some adult input is required to maintain concentration.

Fidgeting

We assess whether the child is displaying abnormally high levels of fidgeting behaviour for his age and if this is affecting his performance.

Case Example

> Anna, aged 3, did not protest at being separated from her parents, but throughout the child assessment was very quiet, immobile, lacking facial expression and maintaining only fleeting eye contact with the clinician. She completed the non-verbal tasks successfully but gave minimal contributions to verbal activities. Such behaviour might be expected initially from a shy child but is not typically maintained throughout a 45-minute period. In Anna's case, the parent interview later revealed that her mother was seriously ill and very preoccupied with her own health, and was also grieving the recent death of her own mother. Anna was confused about the absence of her grandmother, having been told little about her death and not encouraged to grieve, and was perplexed about her mother's behaviour. These issues were central to the remediation process as they underpinned Anna's emotional state, and thereby her fluency.

Cognitive skills

COGNITIVE SKILLS
ORGANISATIONAL SKILLS
DRAWING
PLAY

This section of the assessment is based on observations of the child's approach to various tasks. The data gathered is informal and not standardised but provides valuable insight into the child's general functioning. Any apparent deficits in this area may indicate a referral for detailed assessment to a clinical psychologist or an occupational therapist.

Organisational skills

The two formboard tasks and the wooden abacus provide the opportunity to observe the child's ability to self-organise and problem-solve. The wooden abacus consists of coloured wooden balls which are sorted and placed on graded posts.

These activities vary in level of difficulty and the clinician should record how the child approaches the tasks, making comments about the following:

- The child's ability to structure himself and take logical steps to complete the activity.
- Whether the child visually matches a formboard segment before attempting to place it.
- The child's use of self instruction.
- The child's use of trial and error strategies.
- Whether the child notices and corrects errors.
- The child's readiness to request assistance when in difficulty.

Further observations can be made of the child's manual dexterity and hand preference during these tasks.

Drawing

The child is instructed to draw his mother or father and this picture is scored according to the Goodenough *Draw-A-Man Test* (LDA, 1982). The child is also encouraged to attempt to write his name. Hand preference should again be noted, as well as pencil grasp and any other relevant information, e.g. mirror writing.

Language

Verbal comprehension

Standardised and informal tests are used to assess the child's receptive skills. Test items include commands using objects and picture material as well as tasks with no visual clues, as follows. The therapist gives the instructions and asks the questions as indicated on the form (Figure 2.1) and records the response.

Object material

The child's verbal comprehension is tested, based on information-carrying word levels. Some simple concepts are also tested (see Figure 2.1).

These tasks are based on the *Derbyshire Language Scheme Rapid Screening Test* developed by Masidlover and Knowles (1982). Two-, three- and four-word level tasks are administered and if the child fails on these it is useful to determine if the breakdown has occurred due to auditory memory failure. Establishing when to intervene is problematic, but as a general rule of thumb a 2-year-old child with age-appropriate language skills can be expected to understand at a two-word level, a 3-

OBJECT MATERIAL

TWO-WORD LEVEL

Equipment: brick, spoon, doll, knife, box, plate & cup
Put the knife in the cup ....
Put the brick on the plate ....
Put the doll in the box ....

NEGATION
Equipment: 2 dolls & spoon (place next to one doll)
which doll has no spoon ....
Equipment: 2 dolls, 1 seated & 1 lying
which doll is not sitting ....

DESCRIPTION
Equipment: Dirty & clean doll
Show me the dirty doll ....
Equipment: Wet & dry doll's dress
Show me the wet dress ....

SIZE
Equipment: Big & little spoon, big & little cup
Show me the big spoon ....
Show me the little cup ....

THREE-WORD LEVEL

Equipment: brick, spoon, doll, knife, box, plate & cup
Put the knife under the plate ....
Put the brick in the cup ....
Put the spoon under the box ....
Give me the plate & the spoon ....

FOUR-WORD LEVEL

Equipment: as above + pencil
Put the spoon & knife on the plate ....
Put the pencil in the box & the knife in the cup ....
Put the brick under the box & give me the plate ....
Give me the cup, the brick & the doll ....

Figure 2.1 Verbal comprehension testing.

year-old at a three-word level and a 4-year-old at a four- (information-carrying) word level.

Picture material

The child's comprehension of various syntactic structures is assessed by use of picture material (see Appendix II):

(b) PICTURE MATERIAL

Equipment: Pictures

(i) who isn't sleeping ______

(ii) who is brushing his hair ______

tell me about this one ______

(iii) who has got lots of bricks ______

tell me about this one ______

(iv) who is going to drink the juice ______

tell me about this one ______

(v) who has washed her face ______

(vi) which one am I talking about:

he's playing with a doll ______

she's playing with the car ______

Understanding of negation, tense, plurality and pronouns is tested in order to determine whether the child's comprehension breaks down on specific syntactic items. In addition, the long form of the *British Picture Vocabulary Scales* (BPVS) (Dunn et al., 1982) is administered as specified in the manual to assess the child's receptive vocabulary. This test is particularly useful as it yields standardised score equivalents, percentile ranks and age equivalents. Although this assessment makes no claims to being a comprehensive test of general intelligence it is interesting to note that the BPVS was based on the *Peabody Picture Vocabulary Test—Revised* (PPVT–R) (Dunn and Dunn, 1981) which correlates well with individual intelligence tests. This test result, with information from the cognitive and drawing tasks, will give some indication of general intelligence, concerns about which may prompt a referral to a psychologist for further assessment.

COMPREHENSION WITHOUT VISUAL CLUES

Record child's response

COMMANDS

Open the door & switch on the light..
Stand up & clap your hands ....

QUESTIONS

Why do you brush your hair?...
How did you get here today?..
Where do tigers live?..

CAUSE & EFFECT

What would happen if a wheel fell off a bike? ....
What would you do if a boy hit you?..

DEFINITIONS

Tell me what ... means or Tell me what a ... is

1. hat/chocolate ....
2. running/washing...
3. sticky/hungry ....
4. funny/scared ....
5. disappear/float..

WORD LISTS

Tell me as many animals as you can in one minute
(clothes, types of food). ....
....
....
....
....
....

Figure 2.2 Comprehension without visual clues.

Comprehension without visual clues

A series of verbal commands and questions establish whether the child is able to understand language which is not supported by contextual information (Figure 2.2).

These tasks elicit further information about the child's reasoning skills and expressive language ability. The child is then asked to define a number of words which range from concrete to abstract and the child's responses give indications of both receptive and expressive skills as well as highlighting any word retrieval difficulties.

Finally, the child is instructed to list as many words as possible in a given category, e.g. *'Name as many animals as you can in one minute.'* This task places demands on a number of different skills:

- Comprehension of the instruction.
- Expressive vocabulary.
- Word-finding ability
- Performance under time pressure.

Thus the actual number of words produced is not the only revealing aspect. We are interested in how the child approaches the task: does he systematically label animals category by category, e.g. dog, cat, rabbit, cow, horse, pig, duck, bird, elephant, camel, giraffe? This would indicate an internal structure to the child's lexicon which facilitates retrieval. When the child is trying to think of words, we note 'searching' behaviour as well as increased dysfluency. In addition, we are interested in any evidence of specific word-finding difficulties, e.g. substitution of associated word for target word.

Summary

COMPREHENSION SUMMARY
Length of utterance
Syntactic complexity
Semantic complexity
BPVS score:

The information gathered from the comprehension tasks is then summarised. The receptive level is recorded in terms of how many information-carrying words the child understands in a sentence, as well as levels of syntactic and semantic complexity. The results from the BPVS are also recorded.

Example of completed comprehension summary for John aged 4:2.

Length of utterance:	up to four information-carrying words
Syntactic complexity:	understood plurals, prepositions, and pronouns but not tense markers
Semantic complexity:	difficulty with abstract concepts, e.g. cause and effect
BPVS score:	standardised score 82 age equivalent 3;1 (Chronological age 4;2)

Expressive language

> **<u>EXPRESSIVE LANGUAGE</u>**
>
> Renfrew WFVS: Age equivalent
> Comments
>
> Linguistic analysis
> form
> content
> use
>
> Word finding ability

The child's expressive language ability is assessed by use of the standardised *Word Finding Vocabulary Scales* (WFVS) (Renfrew, 1988) as well as by analysis of language samples from a variety of activities.

Picture naming ability — Word Finding Vocabulary Scales (Renfrew, 1988)

This procedure tests a child's ability to label pictures and the total score may be interpreted into an age equivalent. The test should be administered according to the instruction manual, including the differentiation of failed items into 'does not know picture' (DKP) and 'recognises picture but does not know name' (DKN). Renfrew suggests that if the number of DKN responses exceeds 10% of the total, a specific word-finding difficulty is indicated.

Linguistic analysis

A sample of the child's language output is tape-recorded and transcribed for subsequent analysis. Material should be available for stimulating language. We have found the ***What's Wrong Cards*** (LDA, 1988) to be most useful for eliciting language. The pictures are both humourous and provocative, so that even a 2½-year-old child finds them stimulating. Furthermore, the problem of identifying what is wrong in the picture places demands on the child's naming and word retrieval skills. For example, one picture shows a man ironing with a kettle.

Case Example

> Jane, aged 3;8, responded as follows 'he's doing that, um the clothes, um he's got a tea, a tea pot, um he's ironing the clothes with um, with — what's that'.

In addition, a sample of conversational speech is also recorded and transcribed. When the samples have been orthographically transcribed the therapist is able to undertake a syntactic and pragmatic analysis. This information may then be summarised in terms of the form, content and use of language.

Word finding ability

The child's ability to select an appropriate word from his lexicon may affect his fluency. Any delay in word retrieval will disrupt the child's flow of speech and dysfluent behaviour may emerge in order to fill the pause. During our routine screening of the word finding ability of dysfluent children we have found significantly high numbers of children with specific difficulties in word retrieval. These problems may remain undetected as the dysfluency becomes the main focus of concern; it is therefore essential that any assessment of fluency includes formal or informal tests of word-finding ability.

Wiig and Semel (1984) describe how a word retrieval difficulty may manifest itself in a number of ways. This may include:

- Use of associated words which belong to the same semantic–grammatic class, e.g. 'orange' used as a substitute for 'lemon'.
- Marked delay in naming item.
- Use of circumlocutions and perserverations.
- Increased dysfluency associated with content words.
- Child describes difficulty in retrieving the word, e.g. *'I don't know what it is called', 'I can't remember'*.

In addition, German (1989) includes child's use of gesture in place of the spoken word. The child's word finding ability can be evaluated from his response to other sections of the assessment, such as the tasks without visual clues in the receptive section, in particular the definitions and word lists; the WFVS and the *What's Wrong Cards*.

Any evidence of word finding difficulty will need to be investigated further. If the child is over 5 years old the *Test of Word Finding* (German, 1989) may be administered to obtain standardised data.

Phonology

PHONOLOGY
- intelligibility - delayed/deviant pattern

Conture (1990) suggests that a high number of dysfluent children also have phonological difficulties. It has been our experience that, indeed, some children do manifest such problems although perhaps not as many as the 40% figure that Conture gives. The presence of a phonological problem indicates that the child is at greater risk of stuttering. Therefore the assessment procedure should encompass a screening of phonological development and motor speech processes.

This is undertaken during the course of the whole assessment when any irregularities or substitutions are noted and intelligibility is evaluated. It should be noted whether the phonological deficit is following a delayed or deviant pattern. In the event that a deviant phonological pattern has been noticed a further, more detailed analysis from a transcribed speech sample should be undertaken at a later date, for example, PACS (Grunwell, 1985).

Prosody

PROSODY
- volume
- intonation
- voice quality

During the course of the assessment, aspects of the child's prosodic skills should be evaluated.

The appropriateness of the volume of speech is noted and compared with the parents' volume. We have found that children from larger families often speak very loudly and in some cases voice quality has been affected. This has obvious implications for future management of the child. Furthermore, fluctuations in volume associated with dysfluency should be noticed as some young children increase volume during vowel prolongations, possibly as a strategy to overcome the dysfluency. Similar phenomena have also been noted concerning pitch changes during prolongations. Intonation patterns should also be assessed in terms of whether they seem appropriate to the age of the child. It is rare for a preschool child to be monotonous, but this could be combined with a general lack of affect in a withdrawn child.

Social skills

SOCIAL SKILLS
Observation & eye contact
Listening skills
Turn taking
Position
Facial expression
Gesture

Rustin and Kuhr (1989) describe how the social skills of stutterers may be restricted: 'poor eye contact, impaired listening skills, interrupting and turn-taking, inability to read non-verbal cues, inappropriate body movements and excessive muscular tension during speech'. Thus, these non-verbal behaviours are assessed and judgements made regarding their appropriate use. If social skills are poorly developed or absent, the dysfluent child's verbal ability will appear worse. However, the child with good social skills will be able to communicate more effectively in spite of his dysfluency, e.g. a child who maintains eye contact and normal posture during verbal struggle behaviour will be more engaging than one who looks away and appears to withdraw physically.

Observation and eye contact

Observation skills enable an individual to gather information about people, objects and events in their immediate environment. Fundamental to a child's ability to observe is his use of eye contact. This behaviour is established during early parent–child bonding associated with activities such as feeding a newborn baby. Argyle (1975) states that gaze and mutual gaze play a central role in the development of attachments and sociability. We would therefore expect a preschool child to be using eye contact during interaction with his parents as well as the clinician. In our experience, avoidance of eye gaze due to anxiety, shame or embarrassment, is rare in this age group. An acutely shy child may be reticent to look at a stranger initially, but this is generally shortlived. Aversion of gaze, such as might be a characteristic of an autistic child, would not be expected between a child and his parents. However, we have noted a link between early dysfluency and eye gaze. It has long been acknowledged that many people who stutter have poor eye contact, and this is generally attributed to feelings of self-consciousness about the dysfluency.

Preschool children who show no awareness nor embarrassment about their dysfluency may nonetheless have poor eye contact. Lasalle and Conture (1991) found that mothers of children who stutter gazed more often at their children when they were stuttering, but the children did not gaze back. Conture and Kelly (1991) reported a detailed and objective study of young stutterers' non-speech behaviours. This study indicates that young stutterers produce significantly more non-speech behaviours during stuttered speech than do normally fluent children and produce significantly more head turns left, blinks and upper lip raising. Findings suggest that these behaviours may reflect a variety of cognitive, emotional, linguistic and physical events associated with childhood stuttering. This would support our hypothesis that loss of eye contact may occur when the child is not focused in terms of his thought processes. The eye movements indicate a searching for ideas and language to formulate what the child intends to say. Once these cognitive processes have been harnessed the child focuses visually on his partner in interaction. We have found that improving the child's eye gaze has had a positive effect on fluency. As the child focuses visually and collects his thoughts, he becomes more fluent. It seems necessary for such children to cut off visual distractions and to focus on the person in order to achieve fluency. Detailed research into this area is undoubtedly required, but our initial findings indicate that eye contact affects fluency long before dysfluency affects eye contact.

It should be acknowledged that cultural differences exist in eye gaze norms. Argyle (1975) reports that Arabs have a higher level of gaze than Americans or Europeans, and Japanese look at the neck rather than the eyes. In some cultures eye contact is interpreted as defiance between a child and an authority figure. These variations should be considered when assessing appropriate eye gaze, as it may be necessary to adjust use of eye contact within a family if this will enhance fluency.

Listening skills

Many young dysfluent children present with poor listening ability. This may be due to limited attention control, or to a history of hearing problems often associated with glue ear. Poorly developed listening skills can undermine a child's speech and language development, thereby limiting his capacity for fluency. The child may present as highly distractible, at the mercy of any auditory stimulus. Alternatively, he may be rather self-absorbed, focusing on a single source of input and failing to respond to other signals, as can be observed in a child who is playing with a musical instrument and is completely engrossed in the noise it makes, to the exclusion of listening to any speech or other noises in the immediate environment. Listening skills are fundamental to a child's ability to learn new information, as well as underpinning the capacity to self-monitor.

Turn-taking

Turn-taking behaviour is learned at a very early age. A babbling baby pauses whilst the parent reciprocates in babble, then takes his turn again. Babies learn to take turns in non-verbal activities, such as building a tower of bricks with a parent. Such turn-taking ability relies on observation and listening skills to perceive cues, as well as eye contact to signal it is the other person's turn. Poor turn-taking skills do not often manifest themselves in a one-to-one situation when the clinician assesses the dysfluent child. However, some interrupting behaviour may take place during the assessment or during the parent–child interaction session. Parents may describe a family situation in which turn-taking norms are not being observed, e.g. in a large family children might interrupt one another and their parents and then talk at great length, irrespective of whether anybody is listening.

Position

The child's physical positioning is assessed in terms of proximity, orientation (i.e. angle to the other person) and mobility. Young children often adopt close proximity even with relative strangers but it has been our experience with preschoolers that initially they observe adult-like conventions, becoming more physically involved as rapport is established. The child's level of mobility is also noteworthy. A very active child may have limited attention and listening skills, as well as poor social interaction ability. Alternatively, a very static child might lack the confidence to explore his environment and thus limit his social experience.

Facial expression

We assess how facially animated the child becomes during interaction. Some of the young children we have seen are extremely vivacious and their use of facial expression can be very engaging. There seems to be a wide variation in this non-verbal behaviour, but we have generally found that even if children are not very animated with the clinician, they usually are when interacting with their parents, which will be seen on the video recording.

Gesture

Argyle (1975) found hand gestures to be second in importance to facial cues in the information they convey. The use of gesture in young children varies considerably. However, simple behaviour such as pointing and nodding is usually present. A sophisticated system of gestures may indicate a shortfall in verbal ability or may have developed as a result of a child's severe dysfluency. Many parents have reported a child giving up on a sentence he is struggling with, and resorting instead to non-verbal means of communication, for instance, the child may gesture that he would like a drink.

Dysfluency

Assessment of the child's fluency will determine the nature and severity of the presenting problem, providing the clinician with a baseline measure before treatment. However, dysfluency in young children is widely reported to be episodic and it has been our experience that many preschool children with a severe problem may present fluently in the clinic. On occasions it is therefore not possible to obtain objective, clinically 'clean' data. Instead, we have to rely on anecdotal information from the parents, describing the nature, severity and frequency of the problem. In such cases we encourage parents to make an audio or video recording of the child at home if they have the facility and the opportunity to do so. The quality of this recording will determine whether accurate data can be obtained, but even if it only provides the clinician with an impression of the dysfluency, it nonetheless augments the parental report.

The child's fluency is always measured within the clinical setting even if the parents report it to be better than usual. This assessment is undertaken during a variety of interactions and tasks.

Observation of dysfluency

Firstly, the clinician observes and listens closely during the video recording of the parent–child interaction. The types of dysfluency should be noted and their occurrence in pragmatic categories as well as any apparent avoidance strategies and any facial and body tension.

Transcription

A fluency analysis is carried out on the language sample, recorded during the description of the *What's Wrong Cards* (LDA, 1988) and the child interview. This is transcribed on to the appropriate *Transcription of Dysfluency* sheet in the Child Assessment booklet (see Appendix I). This transcription is augmented by diacritic representation of instances of dysfluency. Phrase repetition and whole-word repetitions may be recorded orthographically. Part-word repetitions, prolongations and struggle behaviour should be represented as follows.

Part-word repetitions

These may be recorded orthographically if the repeated segment is undistorted by the dysfluency, e.g.:

bu bu but

However, if there is evidence of changes in vowel quality, duration or loudness this should be transcribed phonetically. This distinction is made as changes such as these may indicate incipient stuttering behaviour rather than normal non-fluency (Yaruss and Conture, 1993).

Prolonged sounds

These are transcribed phonemically followed by the [:] symbol to indicate length, e.g.:

[m:] ummy
mu[m:]y
m[ʌ:] mmy

Struggle behaviour

For example, blocking of sound accompanied by increased tension should be represented by circling the relevant sounds, e.g.:

(b) all
(a) bout
po(t)ato

We acknowledge that silent struggle behaviour, such as laryngeal blocking, may not be perceptible on an audio recording, so recommend that the clinician makes a note of such behaviour 'live' during the assessment.

When the transcription of the dysfluency is completed, the clinician should listen to the recording once more whilst underlining the episodes of dysfluency on the transcription. Whole-word repetitions should be underlined as one dysfluency, e.g.:

<u>my my my</u> daddy goes <u>to to to to to</u> work = two dysfluent words.

This then reflects the number of dysfluent words in the sample, rather than the number of dysfluencies *per se*.

If the child produces different types of dysfluencies on one word this is also underlined as one dysfluent word, e.g.:

the duck is <u>wə wə w[ɛə:] ring</u> boots.

A short sample from a transcription follows to demonstrate the use of the above techniques:

Example of transcribed sample

That's silly. /bə/ /bə/because the things [a:]re in there. The sock's i i in the cooker. Get h[o:]t and burn. in in a cupboard. The ducks w w w [ɛ:] ring boots. Ducks /də/ /də/ don't wear boots cos they l[ai:]k getting wet. My my my boots are (b)lue He's silly c cos his head [ɪ:]s there and and and his feet are there. Not on the the the pillow thing. [ʃ:]e's writing with a /bə/ /bə/ banana. With a (p)encil. I can write too.

Types of dysfluency

WWR ✔ three repetitions
PWR ✔2–3 repetitions
✔ schwa
PROL ✔3–4 secs
Struggle ✔

17 Dysfluent words (DW)
73 Words spoken (WS)
49 Fluent words spoken (FWS)

Dysfluency measure

When the clinician has completed the transcription the following fluency measures are taken and recorded in the Dysfluency section of the assessment booklet as follows (Figure 2.3).

- Dysfluent words (DW): the total number of dysfluent words should be counted from the written sample.
- Fluent words spoken (FWS): the number of fluent words is then counted from the transcription.
- Total Words spoken (TWS): the total number of words spoken is counted from the written sample. This takes into account all the whole words, both fluent and dysfluent. Parts of words are disregarded. When a whole word is repeated, each repetition is counted separately for this measure (as opposed to the calculation of dysfluent words when several repetitions of the same word are counted as one dysfluent word).
- Length of prolongations: the audio tape is played back and a stopwatch is used to time the length (in seconds) of the longest prolongation.
- Time: two measures of time are taken: (1) Time (seconds) of fluent speech. For this measure dysfluent episodes are disregarded in order to give an assessment of fluent speech rate, which indicates the target rate a child is aiming for; (2) Total time spoken. The total number of seconds is timed for the speech sample, including dysfluent speech. This gives an indication of the child's actual speech rate.

DYSFLUENCY

1. Type WWR no. of repetitions
   PWR no. of repetitions
   PROL length of prolongation
   Struggle
   Other
2. Locus of dysfluency in sentence
   word
   syllable
3. Percentage of dysfluency

$$\frac{DW \times 100}{TWS} = \% DW$$

4. Articulatory rate

$$\frac{FWS \times 60}{Fsecs} = FWS/M$$

5. Actual rate

$$\frac{WS \times 60}{Tsecs} = WS/M$$

6. Occurrence in pragmatic categories

initiation	request	response
interruption	comment	interrupted utterance
imperative		

7. Concomitant facial/body movements
8. Avoidance
9. Awareness

Figure 2.3 The dysfluency section of the Child Assessment booklet.

All the above information is then summarised on to the Child Assessment form as follows (Figure 2.3).

Type

The relevant dysfluent behaviours are ticked and where the dysfluencies characterised by repetitions, the average number of part-word and whole-words are calculated and recorded. The length of prolongations is also recorded here. The 'Other' category may be used to indicate any atypical dysfluent behaviours, such as ingressive airstream or clicks. These dysfluencies should be described and quantified.

Locus of dysfluency in sentence/word/syllable

It should be noted where the dysfluency occurs in the child's speech in terms of the following:

- Position in sentence, e.g. on first word of utterance.
- Nature of dysfluent word, e.g. content word versus function word.
- Position in word, e.g. initial phoneme.
- Position in syllable.

Percentage of dysfluency

A quantitative measure of dysfluency is taken using the data from the sample. The total number of dysfluent words (DW) is divided by the total number of all words spoken (TWS) and this figure is multiplied by 100 to give a calculation of percentage of dysfluent words, as follows:

$$\frac{\text{Dysfluent Words (DW)}}{\text{Total Words Spoken (TWS)}} \times 100 = \text{Percentage Dysfluent Words}$$

For example:

$$\frac{20\ \text{DW}}{363\ \text{TWS}} \times 100 = 5.5\%\ \text{DW}$$

If the parents judge their child's dysfluency to be fairly typical on the assessment occasion, this quantitative measure provides useful data for efficacy studies.

Articulatory rate

A calculation of speech timing is made using the total number of fluent words spoken (FWS) in the sample and the total time of fluent speech (Fsecs), as follows:

$$\frac{\text{Fluent words spoken (FWS)}}{\text{Total seconds of fluent speech}} \times 60 = \text{number of fluent words spoken per minute}$$

For example:

$$\frac{343\ \text{FWS}}{169\ \text{Fsecs}} \times 60 = 121.8\ \text{FWS/M}$$

This provides the clinician with an accurate measure of the child's articulatory rate.

Actual rate

This is a measure of the child's overall rate of output which incorporates the effect of the dysfluency. The total number of whole words — both fluent and dysfluent is counted (TWS) and divided by the total time in seconds (Tsecs) of the child's speech sample:

$$\frac{\text{Words spoken}}{\text{Total seconds}} \times 60 = \text{number of words spoken per minute}$$

For example:

$$\frac{568\ \text{TWS}}{342\ \text{Tsecs}} \times 60 = 99.6\ \text{WS/M}$$

The actual rate of speech may be significantly slower than the articulatory rate. Where this is the case, the calculation of the articulatory rate provides important information about how rapidly the child is attempting to speak, which would not be evident from a measure of actual rate alone.

Occurrence in pragmatic categories

From observation of the parent–child interaction video recording, as well as scanning the transcribed sample, the clinician notes in pragmatic terms when the dysfluency occurs. We are interested in whether the child is more dysfluent when initiating conversation through requests, imperatives or comments. Alternatively, the dysfluency may be more marked when the child is responding to a request or comment by the clinician, i.e. when under some pressure to speak. It is worth noting whether the dysfluency is limited to the child interrupting or being interrupted. It has been our experience that a child's dysfluency may increase when he is in a situation involving competition for a turn to talk, e.g. in a family where several children as well as their parents are involved in a conversation or at nursery/school where children may be competing to have their say. The child is under greater pressure if he has to be opportunistic in interrupting or breaking into a conversation. Having secured a 'turn' he is more likely to speak rapidly, which increases the chance of dysfluency. A further consequence is that the child may then be unwilling to relinquish the limelight and will ramble on while he continues to hold attention. Parents and other adults in this situation may be aware of the imbalance in turn-taking but may be reluctant to stop the child from interrupting or instruct the child to finish for fear of exacerbating the dysfluency. Under these circumstances the dysfluency has 'pay offs' for the child, adding a different dimension to the problem. Thus, it is important to establish whether the dysfluency is linked to turn-taking patterns in the child's environment in order to undertake appropriate management.

Concomitant facial/body movements

Any movements in the face or body which accompany a dysfluent episode, e.g. eye blinking, tongue protrusion, foot tapping, shoulder tension, neck extension, are indications of greater severity as well as potential chronicity if intervention does not take place (Conture and Kelly, 1991). We have found that such behaviour is not uncommon among preschool stutterers, even as young as 2½ years old.

Avoidance

This refers to the child using substitutions or circumlocutions in order to avoid saying a word which might cause dysfluency. The child may begin ***'he's got a cu — cu'*** and then swiftly change to ***'he's got a drink'*** avoiding the word cup.

Awareness

The clinician should evaluate how aware the child is of his dysfluency. This awareness may be manifested during the child interview which is presented below, when the child may actually label and describe the problem. Alternatively, the child may indicate a level of awareness verbally or non-verbally, showing signs of discomfiture or self-consciousness during dysfluency, for example, ***'Have you got a (c)ar — I can't say that word'***.

Child interview — attitudes

This child interview is designed to elicit information directly from the ***child*** about his attitude to nursery/school, home, family and speech (Figure 2.4; see Appendix I). It is undertaken at the end of the fluency assessment when the child is likely to be most relaxed and rapport is established. Open-ended questions should be used in the first instance, for example, ***'Tell me about your nursery?'***. If the child is having difficulty responding then offer some choices. The child's ability to respond to the interview will depend on:

- His receptive language skills — especially when the questions involve higher level abstract concepts.
- His expressive language ability to describe feelings and experiences.
- His concentration span.

Nursery/school

We begin by asking the child if he goes to playgroup/nursery/school (according to age) and whether he likes it. We ask who the teachers are

CHILD INTERVIEW

Nursery/School
- Attitude
- Teachers
- Friends
- What do you do?
- What do you like doing?
- What don't you like doing?
- Teasing — Fights

Home/Family
- Relationship with siblings/parents
- What do you like doing?
- What don't you like doing?

Speech
- Why here?
- How are you getting on with your talking?
- Is it sometimes difficult to talk? — What happens?
- Is it sometimes easy to talk? — When?
- When did it start getting hard?
- Can you help yourself?
- Do you want help?
- How would life be different if no dysfluency?
- Anyone else in family same difficulty?
- Best thing that ever happened to you:
- Worst thing that ever happened to you:
- What do you do when you have problem:
- One change about you:

Figure 2.4 Child interview questions.

and if they are nice/nasty/friendly/cross. It may be appropriate to establish when the teacher gets cross and with whom. We question the child about his friends and what he does at nursery/school. We then ask what he likes and dislikes doing there, which often gives indications of the child's strengths and weaknesses. Teasing, bullying and fighting are also covered in this section, usually in the following manner:

- Are any of the children unkind/nasty/horrible to you at nursery?
- Do they say unkind things/hurt you?
- What do they say/do?
- How do you feel when they do it?
- What do you do when it happens?
- Are you sometimes unkind to other children? What happens?

Home/family

We question the child about his brothers, sisters and parents, asking how they get on together, whether they argue and fight and with whom they like to play. We also ask what they do and do not like to do at home.

Speech

This section is key to establishing how aware the child is of his dysfluency and whether he has an insight into the problem and ways of managing it. This interview is often a very revealing procedure, in that adults often assume young children are unaware of their difficulties. In some households, parental fear of stuttering and a belief that referring to it makes it worse may have rendered the subject unmentionable in the family. However, ignoring the dysfluency does not prevent a child from being aware of it. We have frequently experienced an 'opening of the floodgates' through this line of questioning. It would be inappropriate to put words into a child's mouth, but giving him the opportunity to talk freely about the dysfluency often yields unexpected results. Parents may express fear and concern at the clinician's probing, as well as surprise at the level of the child's awareness, especially when the subject has been so carefully avoided.

We begin by asking the child why he has come to the clinic *'Why did mummy and/or daddy bring you to see me today?'* In our experience, children often reply that they do not know, or that they have come for a day out in London, which may indicate the parents' reluctance to draw the child's attention to any difficulty in speaking. Alternatively, the child might respond that he has come because he 'can't talk properly' or 'stutters'. This may reflect an awareness of the problem, but sometimes it is very superficial — the child is merely repeating what he has been told by others and has no real understanding of what this means. The next question, *'How are you getting on with your talking?'* further probes the child's awareness, followed by *'Is it sometimes hard for you to talk?'*. If the child shows no consciousness of the dysfluency throughout the questions this far, the remaining speech-related questions would be inappropriate. If, however, the child shows that he knows there is a problem, we question further to establish how much insight he has about being dysfluent, what happens and why the problem occurs. *'Is it sometimes hard for you to talk?' 'What happens when it is hard?' 'Why is it hard for you?' 'Is it sometimes easy to talk?' 'When is it easy?'* As before, the child may be responding with information gained from others, which he does not really understand, for instance, *'I can't talk properly because I talk too fast'*. We are interested to establish whether the child has any self-help strategies, and if they are effective, as well as whether he would like someone to help him with the problem. *'Can you help make your speech better?' 'How do you do that?'* The following question, *'How would life be different if you didn't have trouble talking/didn't stammer?'* should be worded using the child's own labels or description of the problem. This abstract reasoning task requires a fairly sophisticated level of receptive linguistic ability and many preschool children cannot cope with it, but the response is helpful in determining the child's motivation and priorities. It is also of value to compare the child's response to that of the parents to the same question at the end of the Parent Interview.

The final speech-related question is asked to determine whether the child is aware of any dysfluency in other family members. *'Do you know anybody else who finds it hard to talk?'* This is particularly interesting if a parent stutters, as we have found some preschool children to be unaware that the parent is experiencing the same difficulty. The four questions at the end of the interview give general information about the child's attitudes and values, his problem-solving strategies and priorities. The final question — *'Let's pretend I can do magic and can change something about you, what would you like me to change?'* — is useful in establishing whether the child is distressed by the dysfluency to such an extent that it is the most important thing to change. A small percentage of the preschool children we have seen replied *'My speech'*. More commonly they say they want to change something about their bedroom/toys/clothes, their appearance as in *'I want to have long hair'*.

Case Example

A child interview was conducted with Laura, aged 3;11, and is transcribed as follows (C = Clinician; L = Laura):

C Do you go to nursery Laura?
L No I go to playschool
C Do you like your playschool?
L Yes, they've got a sandpit there
C You like playing in the sand. I like sand too. But I don't like dressing up.
L I like dressing up but I don't like the trains
C Why not?
L They won't stay on — it keeps breaking
C Is there anything else you don't like doing?
L I don't like colouring. I can't do it in the lines properly — it keeps going over
C What about the grown ups at playschool — do you like them?
L Hazel's nice, she help me do the puzzles
C Is anybody not nice?
L Jane tells me not to walk up the slide but she reads me a story
C What about the other children at playschool?
L Well there's Grant and Edward and Peter — he's naughty cos he keeps biting
C Does he bite you?
L Yes, I cry and Hazel gives me a cuddle

C Who is your friend?
L Edward is. And Lucy and Gemma but not Peter
C Does Peter say nasty things to you?
L Yes he called me a pooh pooh. That's silly talking Hazel says
C How do you feel when he calls you silly things?
L I don't know
C Do you ever say nasty things to him?
L Yes I call him a pooh pooh face
C What happens then?
L Hazel tells me not to be silly
C What about at home. Who is in your house?
L Daddy, Mummy and Tom and Emma and Sam
C Are Tom and Sam your brothers?
L Tom's my brother and Sam is my dog
C Is Tom a big brother or a little brother?
L He's bigger than me. He can push me on the swing
C That's nice. Is Tom ever unkind to you?
L Yes he won't let me play lego and he fights me
C Why?
L He says we pretend to fight but it hurts
C What about Emma?
L She's only one and she cries and spills her drink
C Who do you like to play with?
L I play with Emma: we can roll the ball
C What do you like doing best at home?
L I like my doctors bag and I like my Cinderella video
C What don't you like doing?
L Pretending to fight
C What about your Mummy and Daddy?
L Mummy reads me stories and I'm her helper when she makes a cake
C And Daddy?
L He's at work, I can't be his helper cos I'm not big enough. He swings me round. Not fast though, cos I shout stop
C Why did your mummy and daddy bring you here today Laura?
L I don't know
C I think they brought you here to play and talk with me. How are you getting on with your talking?
L I can't talk all the time. It's hard.
C It's hard to talk sometimes. What happens when it's hard?
L I can't say it. I say a a a
C Why do you say a a a?
L I don't know
C Do you always say a a a?
L Not all the time. Just when it's hard
C Can you stop yourself saying a a a?
L No. I just say it
C Would you like someone to help you with your talking?
L Yes the doctor does an injection
C And that will help you?
L I won't say a a a
C Do you know anyone else who says a a a?
L Uncle Robert does it all the time

C How would your life be different if it wasn't hard to talk?
L I don't know
C Now I want you to think about something. What's the best thing that ever happened to you?
L I don't know
C Somewhere you went, or something you did or when somebody gave you a lovely thing?
L We went to the farm and they had baby lambs and the mummy sheeps didn't like them so I gave them milk in a bottle
C How lovely. Now can you think of something that happened to you that was not nice?
L When I fell off my swing because it was too high. Tom wouldn't stop pushing when I said stop it
C Oh dear did you get hurt?
L Yes, I banged my head and my back but I didn't have a plaster
C Laura what do you do if you have a problem?
L What problem
C When you don't know what to do about something — what do you do?
L I don't know
C Now lets pretend I can do magic and I can change something about you. Anything you like. What would you like me to change?
L Change Tom so he would be a baby
C I see, Tom into a baby. Why?
L Then I would be the big one
C What would you do?
L Nothing. I would be nice big
C What about me using my magic to change you?
L Change me to be very very big
C Why?
L Because I would like that

At the end of the child assessment, after the child and family have left, the clinician completes the assessment schedule, scoring the tests and transcribing the speech sample. This takes approximately 1–1½ hours in preparation for the second assessment session when the clinician will present the results as a part of the formulation at the end of the Parent Interview.

Chapter 3
Assessment of Parent–child Interaction

Introduction

The sample of parent–child interaction is obtained at the beginning of the assessment procedure before any information is exchanged. The clinician explains that it is helpful to obtain information about how children interact with their parents. The parents are asked to sign a form giving consent to the video recording being used for therapy and teaching purposes before the interaction. The parents are each instructed to spend a short time playing with their child whilst being video recorded. They are asked to play as naturally as possible in order to facilitate a typical response from the child and they are instructed not to attempt to make the child talk if he or she seems reluctant to do so. The family is then shown to a room with a variety of play material and the child is invited to choose what he would like to play with and which parent should start the procedure.

The parent–child interaction sample is then video recorded, preferably by use of a remote-controlled video camera and sound system, thereby keeping the effects of intrusion to a minimum. Alternatively, a portable video camera system can be used to record the sample. Parents and therapists are often concerned that their awareness of the camera affects the nature of the interaction. However, research has confirmed our own experience that young children are unselfconscious in the presence of an observer (Lytton and Zwirner, 1975) and parental behaviour remains undistorted (Schulman, Shoemaker and Moelis, 1962).

The interaction sample should be approximately 15 minutes in length and, in keeping with research findings (Girolametto, 1988), the initial and final parts of each recording should be disregarded. Analysis of interaction is therefore focused on the middle section.

The assessment is mainly concerned with the parents' behaviour because therapy will be aimed at helping the parent make changes which will facilitate the child's fluency. However, this should not be interpreted as an indication that we believe the parents' interactive style has caused the dysfluency. We are merely identifying patterns which may be perpetuating the problem or hindering its remission. It is also important to acknowledge here the bidirectional influences during parent–child interaction. A child may affect the way a parent behaves, as well as a parent influencing the child's performance. For example, a passive child will usually compel an adult into a more dominant style. Alternatively, if a parent is highly directive, issuing instructions and controlling the play, the child is likely to become quieter and less active in play. It is interesting to note if and how a child's interaction differs with each parent. Bell and Harper (1977) describe a 'transactional theory' which proposes a bidirectional pattern of interaction in which either partner may influence the behaviour of the other. Lamb and Easterbrooks (1981) state that children affect mothers as well as mothers affecting children. Meyers (1991) discusses the bidirectional process between the listener and the stutterer, and the development, persistence and maintenance of stuttering.

Interaction analysis

This is accomplished by use of the *Interaction Profile* (see Figure 3.1), which is based on the *Interaction Profile* of Kelman and Schneider (1994) and was developed while working with children with language impairment. The clinician watches the video recording of the parent–child play session a minimum of three times, the first viewing for orientation purposes, the second to observe non-verbal behaviours and the third to note verbal interactions. The *Interaction Profile* can then be completed; clinicians should record their observations indicating whether the parents' behaviour is appropriate or inappropriate for the child and the play situation.

Directiveness/following child's leads

This refers to the parents' verbal and non-verbal ability to participate in the play without becoming over-directive or, conversely, taking too passive a role. Observation and listening skills are involved in picking up the child's cues and responding appropriately. An over-directive parent may dominate the play verbally, using too many imperatives and requests, commenting little and giving the child inadequate time to respond, e.g. ***'Right what shall we do with this. I'll put the pigs in this field and you make the other fences. No you need to put it this way up, like I have. Shall I help you? Here I'll do it while you get the other things out'.***

An under-directive parent may make half-hearted attempts to participate in the interaction, taking too passive a role. As previously discussed,

INTERACTION PROFILE

NON-VERBAL		VERBAL
	Directiveness	
	Following child's leads	
		Turn-taking
Listening		Balance of conversation
		Interrupting
	Giving time to respond	
	Pausing	
Gaining child's attention		Rate
		Intelligibility
Observation		Volume
Eye contact with child		Fluency
Shared focus of attention		Prosody
Facial expression		Complexity: syntactic
Animation		semantic
Intrigue		Semantic contingency
Touch		
Gesture		Initiation -
		questions
		– requests
		– imperatives
Position		– comments
– level		– other
– mobility		
– orientation		Commenting
– proximity		Responding
		Repetition
Manner		Rephrasing
– warmth		Maintaining topic
– attachment	Reinforcement	Repair
	Conflict management	
	Choice of activity	
	Response to dysfluency	

Figure 3.1 The *Interaction Profile* (after Kelman and Schneider, 1994); see Appendix I.

parental directiveness is sometimes a function of the child's behaviour, but it is nevertheless an important focus for assessment and treatment. Andronico and Blake (1971) found that training parents in non-directive play sessions with their stuttering children helped increase their fluency. It seems likely that an over-directive parent places greater pressure on the child to perform and communicate during play, thus increasing dysfluency. It is important, therefore, to observe parental directiveness carefully in the interaction assessment.

Listening

We are interested in how well the parents listen to what the child is saying during play. In our experience parents of dysfluent children often report that they have become accustomed to listening to *how* the child is speaking rather than to the actual verbal content. Appropriate listening behaviour is demonstrated both non-verbally, for instance, the parents' position, posture and facial expression, and verbally, for example, following the child's lead, commenting, responding, or maintaining the topic.

Giving time to respond/pausing

This refers to the amount of time parents allow for the child to respond to a question, comment or imperative. We have noted that it is common for a parent to ask a small child a string of questions without pausing for the child's response, e.g. *'What are you going to do with the car?' 'Is it going in there?' 'Do you think it needs some petrol?'* The importance of adequate pausing to facilitate fluency was demonstrated in a study by Newman and Smit (1989). They varied the response time latency in adults and observed the effects on children's pausing and fluency. If the adult responded quickly to a child then the child would, in turn, use a shorter response time. If the adult waited 3 seconds before responding, the child would also increase his response time. Furthermore, two of the four children in the study showed more dysfluency when the adult's response time latency was decreased. Thus, the adult's pausing behaviour is important both in terms of the actual time the child is given to respond, as well as the model provided for the child in pausing before responding.

Gaining child's attention

We are interested in the parents' ability to gain and maintain the child's attention. During play, the child's interest is generally channelled towards the toys or materials with occasional shifts of focus to the adult. However, some children may be highly inattentive, distracted by any sounds or movement in the surrounding environment. Alternatively, many children become so engrossed in the play material that they cut off from any adult interaction, effectively forcing the parent to merely observe or play independently. If the child is either distractible or self-absorbed the parent will need to adopt strategies to gain the child's attention. These include verbal behaviours, such as calling the child's name, as well as non-verbal strategies, e.g. use of touch, positioning and eye contact.

Observation, eye contact, shared focus

We assess the parents' observation skills during the child's play: are they picking up non-verbal cues from the child or have they become engrossed in their own activity. We also monitor the parents' eye contact with the child, noting whether they look when the child is speaking. If they are playing on the floor or if the play material involves intricate assembly, mutual gaze is less likely. In these instances there should be a shared focus of visual attention with occasional fleeting eye contact. Lasalle and Conture (1991) found that mothers of stutterers gazed more often at their children when they were stuttering but the children did not gaze back. It may necessary for the parent to develop strategies to engage the child and re-establish eye contact.

Facial expression, animation, intrigue

We note how much facial expression the parent uses, taking into account cultural differences. This non-verbal behaviour will convey how interested the parent is in the activity as well as providing positive or negative reinforcement. Animation and intrigue also reflect the parents' ability to become involved in imaginative play and to function in a way that engages the child, e.g. adopting different voices for the play characters, using an element of surprise or mystery. Such tactics are useful for gaining a child's attention or refocusing a distractible child.

Touch and gesture

We observe how much and in what way the parent touches the child during play. This may reflect the warmth and intimacy between parent and child. However, the use of touch may convey a tension surrounding the parent's attempts to control the child's behaviour, e.g. if the parent is trying to gain the child's attention is a hand placed on the child's arm or is the arm gripped intensely? The use of gesture augments a verbal message and further engages a child's interest. This may be restricted to pointing or may involve a more sophisticated system of hand movements.

Position: level, mobility, orientation, proximity

We assess the parents' positioning during the play session with the child, noting first whether they move to the child's physical level. This will reflect how involved the parent has become in the play. Parents tend to be more successful in engaging the child if they adopt a similar posture to the child, e.g. children will often lie stretched out on the floor when playing with cars and if the parent follows suit they are more likely to be included in the activity. If the play is taking place whilst seated at a table, it is worth noting whether the parents attempt to bend down so that their head is level with the child's.

The parents' mobility during play is also observed: do they move around with the child or remain static despite the child's movements. This may be more difficult with a highly active child, but if a parent does not follow the child this may reflect an 'opting out' of the play.

Orientation refers to the position of the parents in relation to the child: are they facing one another, playing alongside each other or at a right angle. Again, this will affect the parents' ability to engage the self-absorbed or distractible child.

We also note the parents' proximity to the child: whether they are too close and 'crowding' the child, limiting mobility and self-expression or whether the distance maintained is too great, failing to show an involvement in the activity.

Manner: warmth, attachment

Based upon observation of the parents' non-verbal and verbal behaviour, we record their manner towards the child. Warmth and attachment may be reflected in facial expression, touch and positioning. Parents may appear rather abrupt and detached and it is worth noting this behaviour in order to determine if it is restricted to the artificial play session in the clinic, or whether the parent–child relationship generally lacks warmth.

Reinforcement

This refers to the parents' behaviour in response to what the child does and says. We are interested in whether the parents acknowledge their child's actions, comments or questions and whether they react in a positive or negative manner. Reinforcing behaviours may be verbal or non-verbal, e.g. facial expression and touch. Kasprisin-Burrelli, Egolf and Shames (1972) found that parents of children who stutter demonstrated more negative critical interactions with their children than did parents of non-stutterers.

Conflict management

If conflict should arise during the play session we note how the parents manage this, how the child reacts and the outcome of the situation. This may provide an interesting insight into the parents' handling of challenging behaviour; however, it must be acknowledged that their management of a situation whilst being video recorded may differ from what happens in the home.

Choice of activity

Although the child has selected the play material we are interested in how the parents respond to the situation. A child who chooses cars and a road playmat would often enact traffic scenes or set up a race. However, we have observed parents who use this opportunity for counting and naming colours. Parents may often use a play situation as an opportunity to teach a child, rather than just enjoy the fun of the activity. Alternatively, a parent may set up play at a level too sophisticated for the child, for instance, a parent playing with the child and a teaset may develop the play into a restaurant scenario.

Response to dysfluency

We observe how the parents react to any episodes of dysfluency. Their reactions may be verbal, for instance, instructing the child to 'take it slowly', 'calm down', or finishing the sentence for the child. Alternatively, it may be non-verbal, such as a frozen posture and facial expression, fixing or avoiding eye contact, or tension. Most of these responses will be automatic and unconscious and the parents may be unaware of them until they observe themselves on the video later in therapy.

Turn-taking, balance of conversation, interruption

This refers to the verbal exchange between parent and child. We record whether this is a balanced, reciprocal, to and fro process or whether it is dominated by one party. We also note if the parent is interrupting the child's speech and when and how this is happening. Meyers and Freeman (1985b) found that mothers interrupted their child's fluency failures. They also found that when a child was dysfluent, mothers interrupted frequently, whereas when a child was fluent, mothers interrupted minimally. Mordecai (1979) found that parents of preschool children who stutter interrupted frequently, not allowing their children to answer questions.

Rate of speech

The rate of the parents' speech is measured by timing the parents' verbal output, counting the number of words spoken, and calculating the rate of words spoken per minute. Conture (1990) suggested that a rate of 190–200 words per minute or faster may affect the child's fluency levels. The parents' rate may also be compared to the child's rate of speech: our experience seems to indicate that it is the size of the discrepancy between the adult and child rate which is significant, rather than the actual rates *per se*. Starkweather, Gottwald and Halfond (1990) suggest a rule of thumb that parents' speech tends to exceed a child's rate by about one syllable per second.

Starkweather (1987) noted that an increase in rate was one kind of parental reaction to instances of stuttering. A study by Meyers and Freeman (1985c) found that adults speak faster to children who stutter. We therefore need to consider whether the parents' speech is excessively rapid when compared to the child and thereby increases the possibility of dysfluency.

In some instances the parents' rate of speech may not be unusually rapid but the assessment of the child has revealed a high articulatory rate.

In order to encourage the child to slow down it will be necessary to help the parent reduce their own rate. Stephenson-Opsal and Bernstein Ratner (1988) demonstrated that a reduction in maternal speech rate resulted in a substantial decrease in the dysfluencies of children who stutter.

Intelligibility

We note how clear the parents' speech is, both in terms of intelligibility for the child and as a model for the child's own speech output. We have found that excessively rapid rate, low volume and mumbling may affect intelligibility and on occasions parents have confessed that they are unable to understand their own speech when watching themselves on the video recording.

Volume

We assess the appropriateness of the volume of the parents' speech. If they are too quiet this may restrict their impact on the child's activity, and excessively loud speech may accompany attempts to direct or dominate the session. We have noticed that if a child speaks loudly, perhaps as a part of the dysfluency pattern, parents often unconsciously raise their volume. It should be noted that a sound recording system may distort volume levels as the microphone compensates for loud noises by suppressing the following speech or noises. It is therefore helpful to note parents' speech volume 'live'.

Fluency

The parents' own fluency levels are noted, the types and amount of dysfluency are informally assessed from the video recording and during the parental interview. Parents who stutter may be highly fluent in their interaction with their child, but if this is not the case it is interesting to note if the communication between parent and child is disrupted by the parent's dysfluency. We have sometimes observed high levels of dysfluency in parents who do not consider themselves to be people who stutter. Furthermore, the general pattern of a parent's speech may lack fluency and coherence, being disjointed, circumlocutive and fragmented, a pattern which might then be reflected in the child's verbal output. We are becoming increasingly aware of the wide variety of communication styles to which a child may be exposed and the effects these may have on a child's developing system. Perhaps these children inherit more from their parents than simply a predisposition for dysfluency.

Prosody

This refers to the parents' use of stress and intonation in their verbal interactions with their child. It links with the non-verbal aspects of animation and results in behaviour which may specifically engage a younger or distractible child. We have occasionally observed parents who use inappropriately exaggerated intonation patterns which would be better suited to a younger child. Similarly, very flat intonation may be the first indication of a parent who is suffering some form of depression, an observation that will require validation during the parent interview.

Complexity of language input

The level of semantic and syntactic complexity of the parents' language should be evaluated in the light of the child's linguistic abilities. If the child has receptive language difficulties it is most important that the parents' verbal input is at an appropriate level for the child. Even a child with age-appropriate or above-average comprehension might be placed under pressure by an adult using language beyond his linguistic competence. Conture suggests that 'complex vocabulary/linguistic structures that are too sophisticated for the child's level of development may exacerbate, aggravate, perpetuate or worsen the child's dysfluencies and/or make it difficult for the child to maintain and/or become more fluent' (Conture, 1990, p. 80). There is an increasing body of evidence suggesting that length of utterance is at least as important as complexity in determining stuttering (Gaines, Runyan and Meyers, 1991; Weiss and Zebrowski, 1992; Logan and Conture, 1995). Monitoring the relative lengths of children's and parents' utterances may provide evidence of additional stresses to the child's developing linguistic system.

An adult using long sentences and complex language presents a model which the child may try to emulate. The child attempts to match the adult model and this may precipitate a breakdown in fluency. Haynes and Hood (1978) demonstrated that fluent children show more dysfluency when producing modelled sentences of greater syntactic complexity. It has been our experience that parents of 'only' children commonly present sophisticated models of language with long sentences which places considerable demands on the child's speech output.

Semantic contingency

This refers to the parents' ability to follow the child's intended meaning. We are interested in the relevance of the parents' linguistic input to the child's verbal and non-verbal behaviour. We record whether the parent is speaking in the 'here and now' about what the child is doing with the play material. Parents' responses to a child's speech or actions may be irrelevant or diversifying, or they may attempt to discuss events that are unrelated to the current activity.

Initiation

This refers to the pragmatic nature of the parents' linguistic input. We are interested in whether the parent or child is initiating the conversation, and the form and frequency which these initiations take.

Questions

Questions or requests are common forms of parental initiations. Broen (1972) demonstrated that questions comprise a large proportion of parents' conversational repertoires with their young, normally developing children. Furthermore, Langlois, Hanrahan and Inouye (1986) noted that mothers of children who stutter are more likely to ask their children questions, which is likely to place the child in a position of increased communicative pressure. Mordecai (1979) found that when parents asked their child a question they tended to interrupt the child with another question or statement before the child responded. However, a study by Weiss and Zebrowski (1992) found that stutterers, responses to their parents, requests were less likely to contain dysfluencies than were their assertions. This raises the issue of the different types of questions or requests used by parents. Stocker and Usprich (1976) outlined five levels of demand imposed by questions:

- Level 1 questions produce single-word responses that repeat one of the words in the question, e.g. *'Is that big or little?'* or yes/no questions.
- Level 2 questions produce single-word responses — the name of a common object present but not given in the question, e.g. *'What is it?'*.
- Level 3 questions produce a response consisting of a prepositional phrase where the references are not present and not named in the request, e.g. *'Where would you keep one?'*.
- Level 4 questions produce a series of attributes not named in the request, e.g. *'Tell me what you know about it?'*, 'why' and 'how' questions.
- Level 5 questions are open-ended, e.g. *'Make up a story about it'*.

It is clearly the higher-level questions, demanding a more sophisticated abstract response, which would place greatest pressure on the child's fluency skills. These types of questions or requests are therefore noted. A further point to note is Wood's (1986) observation that questions do not facilitate verbal exchange as much as commenting, thus a parent who is attempting to engage a child verbally by asking questions is using an inappropriate strategy and is likely to be more successful if encouraged to comment.

Imperatives

We are interested in whether the parent is using imperatives or commands to initiate interaction. An over-directive parent typically uses lots of imperatives to instruct the child throughout the activity, thereby controlling the session. Langlois, Hanrahan and Inouye (1986) found that mothers of children who stutter made more demands (imperatives) of their children than did the mothers of fluent children. They suggest this increases communicative pressure on the child, thereby adversely affecting fluency, for example:

Child:	here's a slide.
Parent:	put it next to the swings and put the boy on it. No sit him down. There. Now see if you can find a seesaw.

Comments

Parental commenting may function as an initiation or as a response to a child's utterance. The comment may refer to either the parents' or the child's activity, e.g. *'I'm putting my plate here'*, or *'You have got a blue car'*. Alternatively, a comment may follow a remark from a child, for example:

Child:	I can't put the teddy's coat on
Parent:	I think you've got it the wrong way round.

Mordecai (1979) found that parents of stutterers commented less frequently on the semantic content of their child's utterances than did parents of non-stutterers. Appropriate commenting behaviour involves careful observation and listening and an ability to follow the child's lead.

Responding, repetition, rephrasing

This refers to the parents' verbal behaviour following a child's initiation. We assess whether the parent is responding to the child's questions, requests, commands or comments. Repetition and rephrasing the child's utterances are language facilitation strategies and also serve to confirm the child's intended meaning, for example:

Child:	the boy fall down.
Parent:	yes the boy has fallen off the swing and hurt his leg.

The absence of the facilitative strategies is particularly worth noting in children who have linguistic difficulties as these will need to be incorporated in the remediation programme.

Maintaining topic and repair

Topic maintenance is the parents' ability to continue the theme of the verbal or non-verbal activity. Parents may have their own 'agenda' in play, and prefer to refocus the child rather than follow the child's choice. Repair is the strategy used when the line of communication breaks down due to unintelligibility, dysfluency, or lack of linguistic competence. A parent may choose to allow the subject to 'die' or repair the breakdown by asking the child to repeat or clarify or by attempting to continue the theme through guesswork. If dysfluency is resulting in regular breakdowns in the verbal interaction, a parent's ability to use a repair strategy is particularly relevant.

Selection of interaction therapy goals

When the *Interaction Profile* has been completed (see Figures 3.2 and 3.3) the clinician will need to select and prioritise those aspects of parental style which may become targets for intervention. The items on the profile are not discrete and separate behaviours, they are part of a complex dynamic and bidirectional matrix, each item affecting other aspects of verbal and non-verbal interactional styles.

It is therefore necessary to consider what effect a change in one behaviour would have on others, for example; if a parent who speaks rapidly, using few pauses and giving the child little time to initiate or respond reduces their rate of speech, an increase in pausing may occur thereby increasing initiation opportunities for the child.

The clinician will therefore find it helpful to identify key areas for change as these will form the framework for interaction therapy. The therapist can then help the parents identify their own targets for change, based on the parents' observations of their behaviour. This procedure will be fully described in Chapter 6.

Case Example

Edward, aged 2;11, attended with both his parents. He chose to play with the farm and animals and asked his father to play with him first. We have transcribed the ensuing interaction in order to demonstrate how the *Interaction Profile* is completed.

Father: (lying down on floor alongside Edward and picking up some fence sections). Here let's make fields for the animals. We need to link these pieces of fence together and then we can sort out the animals. You put those fences together (gesturing) and I'll do these.

Edward: (picks up fence sections and attempts to assemble, but cannot do so, discards fence and picks up a cow). This cow hasn't got any eyes. Where's his eyes daddy?

Father: Do you want to put him in this field and find the rest of the cows. I'll make some more fences into fields for the sheep and horses. That's right (as Edward places the cow in the field) now what about the others.

Edward: (picks up two pigs) Where do these go? (places in field with cow).

Father: No not in there. Pigs live separately from cows, they live in a pig sty. Hang on a minute and we'll make one. Oh look I've found a stable for the horses, can you see where all the horses are, and the foals.

Edward: (finds a horse and gives it to his father) Here is one, he's the daddy horse.

Father: That's a stallion, the mummy horse is the mare and the baby is a foal.

Edward: I've found a fold

Father: Not a fold — a foal. Can you say foal?

Edward: Foal. (picks up farmer) here's a man

Father: He's the farmer who looks after all the animals (adopts rustic accent) Now then where's all my horses. I must get them into their field.

Edward: (smiling) Here you are farmer I'll help you catch the horses.

Father: Whoah look he's trying to escape come back you naughty horse.

Edward: (giggling) He's run away.

This play session continued until they were asked to stop so that Edward could play with his mother.

The completed interaction profile (in Figure 3.2) indicates two main areas for intervention:

- Reducing directiveness: encouraging father to follow Edward's leads, observing and listening closely and commenting on his play. This should automatically balance the turn-taking and reduce the level of linguistic complexity.
- Reduce rate of speech and increase pausing.

Mother: (enters room holding a cup of coffee, kneels down on the floor slightly behind where Edward is playing with the animals, placing her drink on the floor next to her). What have you been doing with Daddy?

Edward: no response, continues play.

Mother: Are you going to put all the cows in that cowshed? Is it time for them to be milked?

Edward: They're going inside because it's raining.

Mother: Do you think they don't want to get wet? Maybe they don't mind the rain. We got really wet when we went to the zoo, didn't we? And we had no umbrellas. What animals did you like the best, there.

Edward: This cow is feeling poorly.

Mother: Oh dear what's wrong?

Edward: Well he's got a tummy ache and he's hurt his leg.

Mother: How did he do that?

Edward: He fell over.

Mother: Do you think we should call the vet?

Edward: What's the vet.

Mother: He's the animal doctor. He can make the cow better.

Edward: here's the doctor. Hello cow what's the matter with you.

Mother: (picking up cow) I've got a sore tummy and a bad leg. Can you make me better?

Edward: I've got medicine and a plaster.

This completed profile indicates three main areas for intervention:

- Increase physical involvement in play by encouraging mother to imitate Edward's activity. This should improve positioning and manner.
- Reduce questions and increase commenting.
- Reduce complexity and encourage semantic contingency.

Summary

We have described a procedure for assessing the patterns of verbal and non-verbal interaction between a parent and child. We have also indicated findings from the literature which link interactional styles with a child's fluency.

Having undertaken this assessment and completed the *Interaction Profile*, the clinician is able to identify areas for intervention in the treatment programme which is described in Chapter 6.

INTERACTION PROFILE

NON-VERBAL		VERBAL
	Directiveness *overdirective*	
	Following child's leads *inadequate*	
		Turn-taking *dominated*
Listening *inadequate*		**Balance of conversation**
		Interrupting *some*
	Giving time to respond *inadequate*	
	Pausing *inadequate*	
Gaining child's attention *few non verbal attempts*		**Rate** *rapid*
		Intelligibility *good*
Observation *inadequate*		**Volume** *loud*
Eye contact with child *limited*		**Fluency** *good*
Shared focus of attention *sometimes*		**Prosody** *appropriate*
Facial expression *good*		**Complexity:**
		syntactic } *occasionally*
		semantic } *too high level*
Animation *excellent*		**Semantic contingency** *occasionally inappropriate*
Intrigue *some*		
Touch *appropriate*		**Initiation**
Gesture *appropriate*		**questions/ requests** *some*
		– imperatives *too many*
Position		**– comments** *inadequate*
– level		**– other**
– mobility		
– orientation *(level, mobility, orientation, proximity: appropriate)*		**Commenting** *inadequate*
– proximity		**Responding**
		Repetition
		Rephrasing
Manner		**Maintaining topic**
– warmth *(warmth, attachment: appropriate)*		**Repair** *(Responding, Repetition, Rephrasing, Maintaining topic, Repair: appropriate)*
– attachment		
	Reinforcement	
	Conflict management *N/A*	
	Choice of activity *parents choice*	
	Response to dysfluency *no reaction*	

Figure 3.2 Completed *Interaction Profile* — **Father.** Clinician's comments are in italics.

INTERACTION PROFILE

NON-VERBAL | **VERBAL**

Directiveness *appropriate*
Following child's leads
inadequate non-verbally **Turn-taking**

Listening *appropriate*

Balance of conversation
Interrupting *no*

Giving time to respond
Pausing

Gaining child's attention
no non-verbal attempts
Observation *good*
Eye contact with child *limited*
Shared focus of attention *yes*

Rate *appropriate*
Intelligibility *clear*
Volume *appropriate*
Fluency *good*
Prosody *appropriate*

Facial expression *limited*
Animation *inadequate*
Intrigue *none*
Touch *none*
Gesture *none*

Complexity:
syntactic ⎤
semantic ⎦ *too complex*
Semantic contingency
inappropriate at times
Initiation questions/requests
too many
– **imperatives** *few*
– **comments** *inadequate*
– **other**

Position
– **level** *above child's level*
– **mobility** *static*
– **orientation** *behind child*
– **proximity** *appropriate*

Manner
– **warmth** *abrupt at times*
– **attachment** *rather detached*

Commenting *inadequate*
Responding ⎤
Repetition ⎥
Rephrasing ⎥ —*appropriate*
Maintaining ⎥
topic ⎦

Reinforcement Repair
Conflict management *N/A*
Choice of activity *not physically involved*
Response to dysfluency *some body tension*

Figure 3.3 Completed *Interaction Profile* — **Mother**. Clinician's comments are in italics.

Chapter 4
The Parent Interview

Introduction

Understanding the nature of the family dynamics is an essential prerequisite to our therapeutic intervention. In particular, we need to identify the role the dysfluency plays within the family system. De Shazer (1982) states that once a therapist has understood the ways in which family members view the problem, much more effective suggestions for change can be made. The parental interview is the means by which we seek the parents' perceptions of a wide range of issues. On completion the clinician is able to present a formulation of the problem to the parents and then make recommendations for remediation.

Rustin's *Assessment and Therapy Programme for Dysfluent Children* (Rustin, 1987) included an interview for parents of 7–14-year-olds. During the process of adapting this interview for the younger dysfluent child, many alterations and additions have been made to take account of the developmental and behavioural issues that are of particular relevance to this younger age group. The final version of this parental interview can be found in Appendix III.

The purpose of this chapter is to rationalise the place of the interview within the theoretical model we have proposed in Chapter 1 and to explain the inclusion of such a large number of issues. All the questions fall broadly into the four factors discussed in Chapter 1:

- **Physiological**: questions related to the physiological/neurological predispositions and history of the child, which includes items such as hyperactivity, clumsiness, tics, fits, birth and family history.
- **Linguistic**: anything relevant to the child's speech and language history, including onset and development of dysfluency, current status of speech and language skills, formal and informal assessments of linguistic functioning.

- **Environmental/sociocultural**: this includes factors such as levels of linguistic complexity, child-rearing practices, sibling rivalry, bilingualism.
- **Psychological and emotional factors**: these include the personality characteristics of the child and parents, stressors in the family, such as marital discord or bereavement, and the strategies employed for coping with issues of an emotional nature.

All the questions dispersed throughout the parental interview are designed to help the clinician identify the many variables within each of these factors that put this child at risk of developing a stutter.

The interview

This interview is an active search that will enable the therapist to uncover the many subtle but significant events during the child's development that may be influencing the child's dysfluency and/or recovery. It is a structured interview that has been specifically designed to deal with these issues in a particular order. The first part of the interview allows the parents to talk at length about the dysfluency and its impact on the whole family, and is followed by a history of the child's general health and issues related to child-rearing practices established in the home. A description of the child's personality and communication skills then leads into questions related to intra- and extra-familial relationships. Exploration of the most sensitive and emotional issues concerned with the family history and parental relationships occurs half way through the interview at a time when the parents are most likely to be relaxed and comfortable with the procedure. The interview then returns to more factual information about the birth history, developmental milestones, and the child's sensitivity to change, preparing the parents for the conclusion of the interview. It is important for the therapist to follow this pattern of inquiry asking *all* the questions, as the child's dysfluency could be affected by some or all of these variables. Clinicians may find it helpful to refer to Table 4.1 which has been devised to conceptualise the issues that are most commonly reported by parents and those that are rarely reported as causing concern by this age group. For example, despite recessionary times when unemployment is high, very few parents report financial difficulties; most families seem to be able to manage within the contraints of their circumstances. The issues that appear in the figure as rarely occurring are nonetheless important and should not be omitted. It is only by posing the question that the issue can either be eliminated, or explored until the exact nature of the difficulty has been understood by the clinician.

Table 4.1 Issues most commonly reported by parents of dysfluent children

Most common	*Less common*	*Rarely reported*
Physical health problems	Moving home	Court appearances/police
Family history of stuttering	Clumsiness	Masturbation
Speech and language difficulties	Motor coordination	Difficulties with peer relationships
	Attention disorder	
New siblings	Separation difficulties	School refusal
Loss of grandparents	Parental discord	Parental ill-health
Bereavements	Ill-health of family or extended family	Financial problems
Sibling rivalry		Housing difficulties
Bedtimes — sleeping routines	Custody issues	Employment
Behaviour management	Eating difficulties	Toileting problems
Discipline	Bilingualism	Ritualistic behaviour
Difficulty dealing with feelings or sensitive issues	Families who have a first language other than English	
Personality traits/sensitivity		
	Siblings with other problems	

The inclusion of both parents in the interview procedure is a fundamental principle of our family-based approach. Andrews and Andrews (1990) describe a similar approach to a range of communicative disorders and share our view that:

> Fathers are willing participants when it is clear that their involvement is useful and wanted ... Our efforts to enlist fathers on the treatment team have paid off in benefits to their children, enrichment of our treatment planning, and cohesiveness of the family as the couple engage in mutual decision-making relative to their child.

Our experience has been similar and as a result it has become our policy to make it clear at the time of appointment that both parents must attend and if on the day of appointment they fail we simply renegotiate until a mutually convenient time can be found. It is important, however, to be aware of each family's circumstances so that appropriate arrangements can be made to accommodate them. One-parent families and divorced parents will require a flexible approach depending on the individual situation. We have seen divorced parents together where a good working relationship remains between them. Shared custody and access to the child may make it necessary to interview parents separately when communication has broken down between them. Step-parents and partners that live in the household and take an active part in parenting should also be considered.

Setting the scene

It is important at the onset to establish a comfortable working relationship with the parents, and there are steps the therapist can take that will help to establish a calm professional environment. Collecting all the materials necessary for the assessment and setting up the room so that the interviewer is not behind a desk but facing the parents helps to make parents feel welcome. Simple introductions of all participants, comfortable seating and the offer of refreshments are practical ways of helping parents feel more relaxed before the proceedings begin. Having prepared the physical environment there are also therapeutic skills which may assist the therapist in conducting the interview. It is important to ask questions slowly, simply, directly and clearly and, where possible, to leave them open-ended. The therapist should adopt an unconditionally accepting approach to all the responses the parents make through empathetic listening. It is also helpful at times during the interview to reflect back important information in order to clarify and reinforce that the information has been understood.

Therapists may find themselves being asked for advice or an opinion during the course of the interview and should resist the temptation to begin therapy before the process of assessment is completed. The interview is lengthy but is structured so as to try to minimise the opportunities to become sidetracked. However, therapists should be aware that highly verbal parents wishing to unburden themselves may sometimes need to be drawn back to the interview procedure in order to complete the process in the allocated time. We have found that watching videotape recordings of selected interviews has been an effective way of monitoring and improving our skills in this area.

Introducing the interview

We routinely begin the session by explaining to parents that we need to interview them to ensure that we understand the nature of this child's difficulty within the context of the family, and so that any recommendations will take account of their individual family needs. We continue by assuring them that there are no right or wrong answers to any of the questions and that if there are any questions they do not wish to answer they should say so and their view will be respected. Finally, we comment on the fact that many parents come to the clinician feeling guilty and anxious about the role they may have had in causing the dysfluency. It is important at this early stage to inform them that there is no evidence in the literature that parents are responsible for the onset of their child's dysfluency. However, there is evidence that parents can help them become more fluent. The purpose of these statements is to create an ambience that will encourage parents to verbalise freely in an atmosphere that is positive and non-judgemental. At this point the therapist should begin the interview procedure. It may be helpful for readers to refer to the Parent Interview (Appendix III).

Parent interview

Presenting problem

The therapist should begin by establishing whether there are any other problems apart from the dysfluency that have already been identified by the family, i.e. temper tantrums, difficulties managing bedtimes, slow development, etc. Where there are other problems it is important to ask the parents to indicate how important the dysfluency is in relationship to these other difficulties. Variability is a well documented feature of dysfluency in this younger age group, and parental concern often fluctuates according to the severity of the dysfluency at any given time. Parents of a child who is currently experiencing relatively fluent speech may well find that their attention has become temporarily focused on other aspects of the child's behaviour and this may influence the way in which the therapist will structure therapy for that family.

Case Example

James, aged 3;3, was experiencing a period of relatively fluent speech, when his parents were interviewed. Their anxiety over his speech at that time had significantly decreased. They were, however, very concerned as to how they should manage his uncontrollable temper tantrums. This was taken into account when structuring the therapy sessions for this family and time given to helping them find alternative strategies for dealing with James' behaviour.

It is important for the parents to describe in detail the type of dysfluencies currently occurring. The therapist may find it necessary to assist them in finding evidence of part-word repetitions, whole-word repetitions, prolongations of sounds, or struggle behaviour. This information will reflect the nature of the child's difficulties in the home environment which may be significantly different to the information gathered during the child assessment session. The favourable conditions within the clinic often result in relatively high levels of fluency amongst these children much to the consternation of their parents. It is helpful to ask the parents what they think caused the dysfluency as it will provide important insight into their understanding of dysfluency and their attitude to therapy.

It is important to help parents remember as precisely as they are able the time they first noticed the dysfluency and whether the onset was sudden or gradual, as this has important implications (Yairi, 1992). A gradual onset indicates a developmentally based problem often associated with slower than average speech development, and characterised by relatively easy whole- or part-word repetitions, whereas a sudden onset of dysfluency is often associated with some stressful or emotional event, for example, going to hospital, or starting school. This type of dysfluency is often more severe, with evidence of prolongation and struggle behaviour at an early stage. Questions about how the dysfluency developed and changed after onset and whether there were any major events in the household at that time become relevant to understanding these important issues.

Sometimes families have difficulty recalling the onset of dysfluency and the events surrounding it but as the interview progresses it may become clear that significant events did take place in the family around the time of onset. We may learn of bereavements in or close to the family, moving home or school, illnesses that required hospitalisation, or there may be less dramatic events, such as a playmate moving away from the area, a frightening or painful experience or a series of unconnected and minor upsets. Whilst we cannot be sure to what extent these events are associated with the onset of dysfluency we do feel there may be a cumulative effect on the child which may trigger the emergence of dysfluent speech. The frequency and severity of the dysfluency also need to be established as the degree of variability is considerable and special attention should be given to the context of the dysfluency as it is often highly sensitive to change. An example of this from our clinical experience is the high number of children who appear in the clinic with higher than expected levels of fluency much to the consternation of their parents.

Case Example

Mr and Mrs F came to the clinic with their son, Mark, who was nearly 4 years old and had experienced several periods of dysfluency characterised by long prolongations and struggle behaviour. Mrs F became very anxious during the assessment as Mark was in a relatively fluent phase and was not demonstrating any of the features she was so worried about. She was particularly concerned as this had happened on a previous visit to a professional who advised her not to worry as Mark would probably grow out of it, advice she had found impossible to follow, and which proved unhelpful as Mark continued to have periods of dysfluency which the family found very distressing.

It is important from the beginning to establish with the parents if and how they refer to the dysfluency as they sometimes have strongly held views which the therapist will need to take into account. Many parents have been led to believe that if they ignore the dysfluency, it will go away, a view supported by Johnson's Diagnosogenic Theory (Johnson, 1959). Parents who subscribe to this view often feel very strongly that the child is quite unaware of the difficulty. However, it is our experience that many children *are* aware of their dysfluency and that under these circumstances ignoring it may make it all the more difficult for the child and, indeed, for the parents to cope. It is interesting to speculate that in any other circumstances, if a child had difficulty acquiring a particular skill, the parents' instinctive reaction would be to help. If a child falls while learning to walk,the parent will help physically by offering a support or cognitively by offering advice, such as *'Don't be in such a hurry, slow down a bit'*.

Case Example

> Mrs S, who stammers herself, though mildly these days, was distraught that her daughter, Frances, who was 3 had become dysfluent and was showing signs of struggle. Mrs S was adamant that Frances was unaware of the difficulty and very worried about what might occur if it was mentioned. During our child assessment, Frances was asked *'Tell me about your talking'* to which she replied *'sometimes its really hard'*, *'I go m,m,m mummy like that'*. When asked if anyone else she knew spoke like that she replied *'yes, mummy'*. This little girl seemed relieved to have the opportunity to talk about her problem and ultimately both mother and daughter were able to share something common to both of them rather than continuing to hide an unacknowledged 'dark secret'.

In many cases trying to ignore the dysfluency seems to exacerbate rather than relieve parental anxiety. Furthermore, children who are aware of their difficulties learn very early that the speech difficulty they are having is so unacceptable that it has become one of the unmentionable topics in the household. On one occasion we assessed a family who had developed a code for referring to the stutter. They talked about it as if it was a car, asking after its condition on a regular basis, *'The car has been terrible today, I really think we'll have to get it seen to soon'*. This became even more bizarre when it became apparent that the family did not own a car.

Many parents have already been the recipients of advice from a variety of sources and so it is helpful to know what they have tried to do or say in response to the child's dysfluency. We need to know exactly what each member does and says and whether they, or the child finds it helpful, as parents are often very anxious to know how they should respond and it may be one of the first issues discussed in therapy.

Lastly in this section we need to know how the dysfluency affects the family and how it makes the parents feel. The feelings dysfluency evokes in some parents are considerable and may range from guilt, anxiety, frustration, sadness or pain, to a certainty that the child will grow out of it or finding it 'cute'. It is important to understand parents' feelings about all these issues as it will directly influence their management style. Finally, we need to know of any previous therapy procedures as these may affect the family's attitude to any future intervention.

This first part of the interview has set the scene, allowed the parents to talk at length about the problem as they see it and discuss their feelings about it. It has also allowed the therapist to share the family's experience and beliefs about the dysfluency and the way in which these affect their management of the child.

General health

In this part of the interview questions are asked about the child's physical wellbeing, and any impact this has had on school or home life. The responses given to these questions may also indicate physiological and or neurological factors that will predispose the child to fluency breakdown.

A child who has a history of asthma attacks, has had several episodes in hospital and is described as 'clumsy' presents a very different picture from one who has occasional stomach aches, has had chicken pox and measles, and wears glasses. It is important not only to know about the incidence of illnesses and when they occurred but also to ask how these episodes were managed, the child's response and the effect on the family as a whole. It is important to ask if the child is on any medication and whether there are any side effects. Persistent headaches or stomach aches should be investigated as they may be related to a number of different issues, e.g. dislike of school, diet, stress, a family history of migraine.

We need to know that the child's hearing and sight have been tested and the results of those tests. In small children these factors are of particular relevance due to the high incidence of glue ear and the effect that this has on the child's speech and language development and management. If these have not been adequately dealt with, recommendations may need to be made at the end of the interview.

Attendances at other clinics will give insight into other concerns the family may have regarding this child. If they have attended child guidance, for instance, they may already be concerned about the child's behaviour or their ability to manage certain aspects of their parenting role. It would be important to understand what prompted them to attend and the outcome.

Questions related to concentration, over-activity, facial tics and clumsiness, derive from neuro-psychological theories of dysfluency (Moore and Boberg, 1987) which imply generalised deficits in brain functioning, leading to motor speech impulsivity and lack of neuromotor control (Rosenfield and Nudelman, 1987). The theory suggests that children exhibiting difficulties in these specific areas may be more vulnerable to fluency breakdown. Handedness also falls into this category, it is viewed as a manifestation of cerebral lateralisation with mixed handedness an indication of incomplete or atypical neurological lateralisation.

Behaviour

Eating, sleeping and elimination routines, are especially significant to this younger age group. They are powerful and emotive issues which are often difficult for relatively new parents to deal with satisfactorily. Parents experiencing difficulties in any or all of these areas often feel exhausted, guilty, frustrated and out of control. Coping skills will vary from family to family and therapists will need to understand how parents are managing, as it will inevitably affect other aspects of family life and the relationships between the family members.

Sleeping patterns are of particular relevance as children can very successfully disrupt the household by refusing to go to bed, not going to sleep, waking up many times during the night or sleeping regularly in the parental bed. Furthermore, most parents report that the child's dysfluency increases when they are tired. Mealtimes, toilet training, and bedwetting can also become battlegrounds for parents, each family will have a view about what is acceptable and it is important for therapists to understand this before making recommendations at the conclusion of the interview.

Case Example

Mr and Mrs P had three children, Peter, aged 5, David, aged 3, who was dysfluent, and Katherine who was 2. The two older children shared a bedroom and Katherine, the baby, had a room of her own. Mrs P found bedtime a real trial and had little support from Mr P who did not return home from work until after 8.00 pm. Mrs P attempted to get all the children in bed between 7.00–7.30 but often found it was nearer 8.00 pm. Added to this David often got up in the night to go to the toilet and found his way into the parental bed until morning. The management programme therefore included helping Mr and Mrs P re-structure the bedtime routines and David's nocturnal visits. This subsequently played a significant role in reducing some of the stress within the household.

Communication

This section looks at the parents' awareness of the child's ability to communicate both verbally and non-verbally and gives the therapist an insight into how the child functions outside the clinical setting. This information may also be useful when discussing the results of the child's speech and language assessment with the parents at the conclusion of the interview.

Personality

It is important for each parent to describe the personality characteristics of the child as it will help the therapist understand the child's emotional vulnerability to moments of dysfluency. The child described as 'happy go lucky', 'easygoing' and 'extrovert' will respond very differently to moments of fluency breakdown than a child who is described as 'perfectionist', 'fussy' and 'a worrier'.

In the preschool years children's temper tantrums can cause a great deal of distress to all concerned. Details of the situations and circumstances which provoke these as well as the ways in which each parent deals with them will help the therapist see the dysfluency in the context of a variety of other management issues, which may need to be addressed. Some families successfully manage the tantrums of their fluent children, but find themselves unable to use the same strategies with the dysfluent child, for fear of exacerbating the speech problem.

Some children may have very specific fears, for instance, the dark, dogs, or death; clinicians should explore the antecedents to these, and the way in which they are handled. Many children are fussy about something, commonly their clothes or what they will eat; identifying those who are excessively fussy is important as they are often difficult to manage. Children who display ritualistic behaviour need to have a sequence of behaviours maintained, for instance, lining up the teddies every night in a certain order on the bed before they will get in to the bed; these children also become very distressed when these patterns are disturbed. Truly ritualistic behaviour is an indication of considerable anxiety and insecurity in children and though in our experience it rarely occurs, when it does it should not be overlooked. Although comfort habits are quite common in this age group they are often seen to be indicators of a child's emotional state and need to be noted. The way children separate from their parents, and cope with new experiences will provide further information about how the child is managing the emotional demands that are being made upon him.

Relationship with peers

These questions will elicit the names of some of the child's friends, the preferences they show in age or gender, the role they like to play and whether bullying, teasing or fighting is part of the social milieu in which the child finds himself. Bullying and teasing is always a highly emotive issue for both child and parent and where it occurs it causes great anxiety and distress. For some parents and children helping with these issues may be a priority.

Relationship with siblings

It is important to establish the names and ages of all the siblings and the dysfluent child's position in the family. We need to know how they interact with each other, with whom they play, whether there are any particular attachments and how these are shown. Most siblings squabble but it is helpful to know where the conflicts are and the role jealousy plays amongst them. Finally, we need to know if there are problems with any of the other children in the family as this may be highly significant.

Case Example

The Browns had three children, the eldest, James, was very dysfluent; Sam, the middle child, who was only 20 months younger had a severe behaviour problem which had been evident since he was very young. During the interview it became clear that although the family presented James' dysfluency as the problem, it was in fact Sam's behaviour that was disturbing the equilibrium of the family. The recommendations for this family were focused initially on helping the family seek the help they needed for the management of Sam. Once this was in place it was possible to make progress with James' dysfluency.

Relationship with adults

We ask each of the parents to describe their relationship with the dysfluent child, with respect to the characteristics they both like and dislike. We look at the ways in which family members show affection towards each other and finally find out how the child relates to other adults, e.g. teachers or family friends.

Case Example

Emily was 6 years old, an only child of parents who both worked in the arts and education. Emily was accustomed to adult company and made good relationships with many adults in her environment. She had acquired a very adult vocabulary and linguistic skills several years in advance of her age. However, she had difficulty relating to her peer group and her dysfluency was clearly associated with the problems she encountered establishing herself at school. Helping the parents to understand these issues and how they could help Emily by making changes at home was very important in her eventual recovery.

Sex education

Therapists may have difficulty asking questions about the child's interest in and knowledge of sexual matters. However, children do often ask questions related to these issues and it is helpful to understand how the family will respond as it provides insight into their ability to deal with subjects of a more sensitive and intimate nature. There are those families who are very open and relaxed and deal with these issues as they crop up in a straightforward and easy manner, whereas others have much more difficulty, feel embarrassed, would rather not discuss it, and change the subject. Clinicians should also be aware of, and take into account the differing views of various ethnic minority groups. For example, the Hasidic Jewish community would consider conversations regarding sex highly inappropriate, as discussions of this nature only take place when the child is of a particular age or before his/her marriage. The clinician should also ask parents if the child masturbates. Although it is quite commonplace for small children to play with their genitals, it occasionally becomes a problem and can be a source of considerable concern and embarrassment to a family. It may also be the sort of problem they feel unable to share with anyone or seek advice about. The role of the speech and language therapist here is to understand the nature of the problem and how it affects the family so that appropriate recommendations can be made at the end of the interview.

Case Example

Mr and Mrs F described 5-year-old Louise as a demanding child who talked incessantly. There had been many difficulties in Louise's early development that resulted in her being a frail child for some time causing considerable anxiety to all concerned. When asked questions about masturbating, after a momentary pause, Mr and Mrs F immediately described their concerns about Louise who was touching herself frequently at home and in public. It was causing considerable anxiety and embarrassment and they were beginning to be reluctant to take her out with them. The relief experienced by the parents at being able to unburden themselves was almost palpable. For this child, the behaviour was one of many other difficulties which we felt needed further investigation and appropriate referrals were made as part of the recommendations at the conclusion of the interview.

Schooling

The child's school history may include mother–toddler groups, play groups, nursery school, etc. The dates of attendance and the child's reaction is important information as we have often found that it coincides with the onset of or the exacerbation of the child's dysfluency. The extra demands, the emotional and physical separation and the adjustment to an unfamiliar environment can make a significant impact on the child's fluency. Information from the staff about the child's progress and development and, where appropriate, comments concerning his skills in reading, writing and numeracy will also be helpful. Dysfluent children frequently have co-occurring speech and language difficulties which may be reflected in their reading and writing skills; if these can be identified then much can be done to provide remediation in the early stages of their education.

Family structure and history

The family structure and history is the core of the procedure and has been placed at the centre of the interview to ensure that parents are prepared for the sensitive and probing nature of these questions. First, we need to establish the duration of the parents' marriage or their relationship where there is no formal union between them, and any periods of separation during that time. Previous long-term relationships or marriages are also relevant, especially if there have been children resulting from these. Clinicians should record details of any other children, including their sex and age, and the contact that is maintained between all parties.

Case Example

Mr and Mrs P had two young children, 5-year-old Sarah and 3½-year-old Thomas, who was dysfluent. During the interview Mr P told us of the two teenage children he had as a result of a previous marriage. The children were unaware of each others' existence, despite living in such close proximity that a chance meeting was a possibility. Mr P's desire to maintain this secret was just one example of the difficulty this family had discussing issues of a sensitive or emotional nature, and as a result of the interview could be seen as a well established pattern that had its origins in his own upbringing. Mr P had not experienced a close or intimate relationship with his parents, a fact he regretted. Facilitating discussion between the family members and opening the lines of communication became an important part of the therapy approach. The changes brought about had an immediate effect on the way in which they managed Thomas' dysfluency and a long-term effect on the way the communication system changed within the family.

There is increasing acknowledgement that the experience of miscarriages, stillbirths, and/or terminations should be managed in a similar manner to a death in the family. It is necessary, therefore, to ask questions that will establish the circumstances surrounding these events. Parents may still be deeply upset by a miscarriage, stillbirth or termination. The effect these experiences have on an individual's emotional state cannot be under-estimated and will be highly relevant to the understanding of a particular family's dynamics.

Case Example

Mrs S had several miscarriages before the birth of Tom who was 3½ when he came to see us. Tom had started to be dysfluent at 3 years, at a time when his vocabulary and syntax were expanding at a great rate. Mrs S had had several miscarriges and was devastated by the miscarriage she had immediately before Tom, as she had carried the baby for 4 months before losing it. Mr S had failed to appreciate the intensity of Mrs S's distress, seeing it as 'one of those things' and that they would simply try again. The birth of Tom was greeted with great joy but Mrs S was from the very beginning fearful of losing this precious child. She was very protective of Tom but also held unrealistically high expectations, wishing for him to be the perfect child, to make up for the loss of the others. Helping Mr S understand the difficulties Mrs S experienced in coping with the deaths of the previous children and helping them talk through these experiences with each other, helped them re-look at their management of Tom. Mr S was eventually able to be much more supportive of Mrs S and the consequent improvement in their relationship led to further productive changes in their management of Tom.

In most cases clinicians will be aware of children that are adopted or fostered. However, this is not always the case and it is important, therefore, to request the information. Children are adopted in a variety of ways and under very different circumstances, which may become an issue of special significance and sensitivity. It would be important to understand how the adoption had been arranged and anything relevant to the child's or parents' circumstances prior to adoption. Some families have great difficulty disclosing information regarding adoption preferring to keep the 'secret' within the family. Unfortunately maintaining this 'secret' can in itself create problems which the family needs to address.

Case Example

Mr and Mrs T adopted Lee as a very young baby and had kept their secret for several years. At the time of interview Lee was 4 years old and had become dysfluent at 3 years. They found the interview difficult as they attempted to maintain their silence regarding Lee's adoption. However, during the penultimate section of the interview they were able to discuss the adoption and their concerns for this very 'special' child whom they feared they might lose. The circumstances surrounding the adoption were complex and their fear of losing this child was creating great anxiety and affecting their management of Lee. Discussing these issues openly led them to make decisions that were instrumental in stabilising the family.

Personal background

Gathering information related to the personal and family history of each parent helps us to understand how the current family members are functioning. In addition, knowledge about parental upbringing will provide invaluable insights into their own parenting style.

The age, place of birth and religion of each parent gives us information about their cultural and religious origins. Where these are very diverse it is often helpful to ask how they have reconciled these differences.

The occupations, and educational history of the parents will reveal their experience of school and further education and, moreover, may influence the expectations they may have of their own children.

Health issues are very important in families, a parent with a health problem will affect all other members of the family in a variety of ways. The therapist will need to ask about each parent's general health, any medications they may be taking, and the impact it is perceived as having on the rest of the family.

We ask each parent to describe their personality. For example, *'How would you describe yourself, what sort of person are you?'*. Some parents have difficulty with these questions and may ask their partner to help, the therapist simply redirects the question and asks the partner to wait as it will be their turn next. It is important to allow the parents time to formulate their response, as the insights gained from their descriptions will be invaluable. We have found it useful to reflect back their description thus: *'You describe yourself as "sociable and caring, a bit of a perfectionist and rather moody at times", is there anything else you would like to add?'*. Finally, we ask the partner if there is anything they would like to add to the description, and then repeat the whole procedure with the partner if there is one. This insight into the characteristics of each parent is often crucial to our understanding of the dynamics occurring within families. A mother may describe her child as a worrier and when she ascribes the same characteristic to herself we can begin to appreciate how the one may exacerbate the other. The ensuing questions aim to discover whether either of the parents have had emotional problems, depression, or have seen a psychiatrist. Where the answer is positive, the circumstances and outcome also need to be explored. It is particularly relevant to ask each parent if they have any history of stuttering, even if only briefly during childhood, as this will place their children at risk. Details of any treatment they may have had will give some insight into their expectations of recovery or therapy outcome. For example, a father who has a long history of stuttering and of unsuccessful therapy will have a very different attitude towards therapy than one who stuttered until 13, 'grew out of it' and expects his child to do the same.

Many dysfluent children have other accompanying difficulties so we ask parents to describe any problems they had learning to speak, read, write or spell as these problems often run in families.

Alcohol-related problems can have a devastating effect on families and it is often an issue that is not discussed or may be kept secret. We have found that the most effective way of asking this question is to ask the mother if the father has any alcohol-related problems and vice versa, as it makes it more difficult for a parent to deny it. Where a problem exists, the therapist should ask further questions to establish the nature and extent of the abuse, its affect on the family, and any help they have sought or might require.

The same procedure should be applied to the question relating to drug use. In both cases the effect on family life and relationships is often crippling and making appropriate recommendations may be critical to the future development of the family.

The occurrence of epilepsy in the family history is interesting to note, especially where the dysfluent child is showing signs of a similar pattern emerging.

Finally in this section, we are concerned about any court appearances parents may have had. Therapists often ask the relevance of this, which is perhaps best illustrated by an example.

Case Example

Mr and Mrs C had a son, Dave, who had been dysfluent since he began to talk at 3 years. The parents had not been able to think of significant events that occurred around the time of onset but on being asked if anyone had been to court, the father, after a pause, said that he had been to court after a fight that developed when the car he was driving had broken down in the middle of the street not far from where they lived. The man in the car behind became very angry as he was unable to overtake. An argument ensued culminating in the man picking up a crowbar from the car behind and attacking Mr C through the window of his car. The glass and the crowbar caused serious injuries to Mr C's face. The police were involved and Mr C was able to identify the man in the car, who was subsequently sent to prison for several years. At the time of the interview there was considerable anxiety in the household as the man lived locally, was shortly to be released, and the family had been threatened on several occasions. As the details of these events unfolded, it also became evident that it had coincided with the onset of Dave's dysfluency.

Parents' family background

The questions within this section will enable the therapist to understand how the parents' early life and experience of being parented may have shaped their own child-rearing styles. There is considerable evidence that family patterns and histories tend to repeat themselves, thus an awareness of each parent's experience as a child can be helpful in understanding their current child-rearing practices.

It is important to understand the role the grandparents play within the family. Some grandparents wield considerable power and influence in families, whereas in others there may be little or no contact. In the event that grandparents are deceased full details should be recorded, including their age, the date and cause of death and the circumstances surrounding the event. Therapists need to understand how the parents managed their bereavement and to appreciate that stresses may still exist and be influencing the family dynamics. However, in some cases the children will also have experienced the loss of a grandparent and the therapist should explore how the family managed this situation. Parents who are in a high emotional state often exclude the child from the grieving process, in an attempt to protect them from pain and distress. Ironically, this can cause the young child confusion and feelings of guilt, as he tries to interpret the conflicting messages he is receiving.

Case Example

George, who was 4, had a very close relationship with his grandmother but was told she had gone on holiday when she died. The mother was so distressed herself, she wished to spare George these feelings, not realising that in the long term she was compounding the problem for them both. She would eventually have to tell him the truth and George may learn not to trust her in future.

Extended Family History

This section provides information that will enable the therapist to look at the family patterns, history, and predispositions. It may also provide essential insights into the extended family, for example, discovering a family history of depression may help the therapist see the father's 'moodiness' as part of a familial pattern of depression. Alcohol- or drug-related problems also cause great distress in families and this information will be helpful in the final formulation.

Case Example

Jane, the mother of Joseph aged 5½, had found it very difficult to deal with the death of her brother who was a drug addict. This was still causing Jane a great deal of pain and guilt and resulted in uncontrollable mood swings which affected her management of Joseph. Joseph was unaware of Jane's distress over her brother but very aware of his inability to predict her behaviour a fact which left him feeling insecure and anxious. Once Jane explained the reason behind her mood swings, Joseph ceased to blame himself and became sympathetic to his mother who was sad sometimes because she missed her brother.

Home Circumstances

The questions in this section look at the way in which the physical environment affects family members. The space available, the organisation of the sleeping arrangements, etc. all have a part to play.

Case Example

Keith, aged 3, shared a bedroom with his two older brothers, aged 5 and 7 years, and refused to go to bed until they did; as a result he was constantly tired. Rules regarding bedtime and changes in the sleeping arrangements to allow the children space of their own became important components in the therapy for this family.

Where there are other people sharing the family home, it is important to find out how this affects the dynamics within the home environment. Grandparents, extended family members or even lodgers may at times be helpful, but may also place additional demands on the household and stresses on those relationships.

The therapist should explore the childcare and organisational arrangements, especially where both parents are involved in working outside the home. Details relating to the childminder, nanny, au pair, or nursery, including the child's response to the carer, should be noted and, where appropriate, carers should be incorporated into the therapy programme.

A description of the neighbourhood the family resides in, whether they like it and how long they have lived there, indicates the stability of the physical environment and the likelihood of this continuing in the future. Frequent moves, or an unsuitable home environment can create considerable stresses within families. It is essential for therapists to understand the nature of the difficulties, as in some cases it may be necessary to help the family resolve these before therapy commences.

It is interesting to note that despite recession and high unemployment very few families report having financial difficulties as they seem to adapt to differant financial circumstances. However, where there are serious concerns, the impact on the family may be considerable, and directing the family to an appropriate source of help will need to be discussed at the end of the interview.

Family life and relationships

Understanding the core of the parental relationship and their day-to-day activities is essential as it will profoundly affect the future development of the family and the nature and timing of the therapy that will be recommended. The parents' responses are generally frank and open as the clinician will have maintained a neutral, unconditionally accepting attitude towards the parents throughout the interview. In the event that parents are expressing difficulties in their relationship, therapists should explore the strategies, if any, that they are employing to deal with it. It has frequently been our experience that unresolved issues between the parents' interfere with the process of therapy, especially where the dysfluency has been functioning as a distracter within the family. It will be essential for the therapist to discuss with the parents the relevance of these problems during the formulation at the end of the interview. Offering them some help in addressing the difficulties within their relationship through individual sessions or by referral to outside agencies, such as marital therapy, may well be an important component of their therapy programme.

Further questions about the role the father plays in helping at home, the friends that the couple have, and the manner in which they resolve problems at home, will shed light on the support systems that this family have and how they use them. Parents who are well supported by a network of family and friends living nearby may be much better able to cope than a similar family who have no such system in place and are only able to rely on each other.

Statistically, the number of single-parent families is increasing, thus we have included a series of questions for these circumstances that will help the clinician understand the nature of the relationship between the mother, the child and the father. We wish to understand the manner in which the parents separated, the circumstances, custody and access issues and the effect all this has on the child. The single parent's current relationships may also be relevant, especially if there is a person in the home who plays a role in parenting.

We need to establish the opportunities there are within the family for sharing and participating in child-orientated activities. It is interesting to note whether these activities are confined to one parent or shared between them.

Case Example

> Charlie was a 4-year-old who had a good relationship with his parents but was particularly attached to his father. During the interview it emerged that the father had a very demanding job which took him away from home and he regretted not having more time with Charlie. This was subsequently discussed with the parents during the formulation and a time was negotiated for Charlie and his father to go swimming together once a week. This was one of the first changes that occurred during therapy and was very important for the relationship between the boy and his father.

It is also helpful to know if the child is willing or permitted to help with household chores as this can be an important feature in the parent–child relationship. Mothers who are orderly and perfectionist may have great difficulty allowing their children to help. Assisting them during subsequent therapy sessions to make small changes in their management of these situations can be very productive.

Finally, it is interesting to note in whom the child confides, and whether there are any other adults in the environment to whom they are especially attached.

Antisocial Behaviour and Discipline

Management of young children's behaviour and discipline is often a cause for concern to parents, and the next few questions are directed towards finding out if this is an area of difficulty for the family. The therapist needs to find out precisely what the parents do under these circumstances. What form of discipline they use and, most importantly, if they are consistent and support each other both in what they say and the actions they take. The final questions in this section relate to the rules if any, that apply within a particular family.

Case Example

> Mrs S described her household as chaotic and her children as out of control. She had recently become quite depressed and was finding herself increas-

ingly desperate as the children's behaviour worsened. Mrs S was a single parent and considered having the children taken into care. Helping Mrs S praise her children and establish some simple rules in the household was an essential prerequisite to any recommendations regarding the dysfluency.

Child's developmental history

The child's development history is covered in this section. The questions begin with the usual details of mother's pregnancy and the birth of the child, but we also ask whether this pregnancy was planned and how the child's birth affected the family life style. Sometimes the impact of a new baby is considerable and should be considered.

Case Example

Mrs W recently told us of the shock she had on finding herself pregnant. Mr and Mrs W had talked of having children 'one day' but were not prepared at that moment for the emotional and physical changes they had to make in their lifestyle and employment plans at that time. Although Matthew's birth was uneventful, he 'arrived screaming and never stopped'. Matthew was diagnosed by the doctor as having colic and the early months were dominated by an unsettled baby that cried continuously and slept very little. These circumstances created a great deal of anxiety and stress. The parental relationship deteriorated, and the mother described these early months as 'dreadful'. Matthew continued to be a handful who was prone to regular explosive tantrums which the parents found very difficult to manage. It was very important to help these parents find time for themselves and their relationship, as well as helping them to plan and implement more productive ways of managing Mathew's behaviour.

Separations

It is important to note periods of time that the child has been separated from the parents. These may include hospitalisations for the child or parent, for which the circumstances and the child's reaction should be noted.

Emotional expression/sensitivity

This final section investigates how the child expresses emotions and his sensitivity to situations of an emotional nature. It is also interesting to note how the child's life might be different if he was fluent and also the effect this might have on the parents. It gives considerable insight into the implications there are within the family for a change of this kind. Future impending changes anticipated within the family will also give the therapist warning of events that might affect the family and may influence recommendations made at the end of the interview.

At this point the interview is complete and it is important for the therapist to thank the parents for their help, and to ask them if there is any information they have that has not already been covered. If there is no further information the parents should be advised to take a few minutes' break. During this time the therapist should gather together the information from the assessment of the child, and the parental interview prior to the formulation which is discussed in the following chapter.

Summary

The parental interview provides the framework within which the clinician is able to explore all the subtle but often significant variables that may exacerbate as well as perpetuate the child's dysfluency and or recovery.

The format presented in the interview procedure allows for clinicians to develop their own wording and style when asking questions. Experience suggests that neutral open-ended questions give parents the best opportunity to reply. ***'Tell me about bedtimes' 'What happens at bedtime?' 'How do the children get to bed?'*** allows parents freedom to describe the activity in their own terms as opposed to ***'There aren't any difficulties getting the children into bed are there?'***. It is also important for clinicians to observe the interaction of the parents during the interview to ensure that their verbal and non-verbal behaviour have been understood by the clinician. Clinicians may also find it helpful to seek clarification from parents from time to time by summarising important issues and inviting the parents to check their understanding of the information. Providing all the questions have been asked, at the conclusion of this interview, clinicians will be able to make recommendations for therapy, based on the individual needs of the child and the family.

Chapter 5
The Formulation

This final stage of the full assessment procedure is perhaps the most important, as it is at this point that the clinician is in a position to present a professional view of the problem in a way that is meaningful to the family.

The length of time required to complete the interview will vary, but therapists should anticipate at least 2½–3 hours. Upon completion therapists may need a little time to return to the material gathered during the child assessment. Those unfamiliar with these procedures will also find this time provides an opportunity to assimilate and organise the wealth of material collected before sharing the formulation with the parents. The Summary Chart (Figure 5.1) has been designed to assist in the process of drawing together all the information gathered during the assessments and interviews, focusing on the issues of particular relevance to each individual family. It also reflects the multifactorial model presented in Chapter 1 and provides a framework within which the therapist can make clear the relationship between the theoretical model and the circumstances and events in each family's life and history.

The four factors discussed in Chapter 1: physiological, linguistic, environmental/sociocultural, psychological/emotional are represented on the Summary Chart as a circle, reflecting the dynamic interaction that occurs between them. The chart is then further divided by elements from the case history and the assessments that are most commonly found to be important in the formulation of the problem. Table 2.1 demonstrates where the information is gathered in the various assessments and interviews and can be found in Chapter 2 (p. 15).

The therapist is now in a position to review the interviews and assessments and consider each factor in turn, placing significant items on the Summary Chart. We have found it helpful to begin with physiological and linguistic factors as these give some indications of the child's predisposition to dysfluency, both organic/genetic and linguistic, and then to consider the environmental and emotional demands that are being made on this child's system.

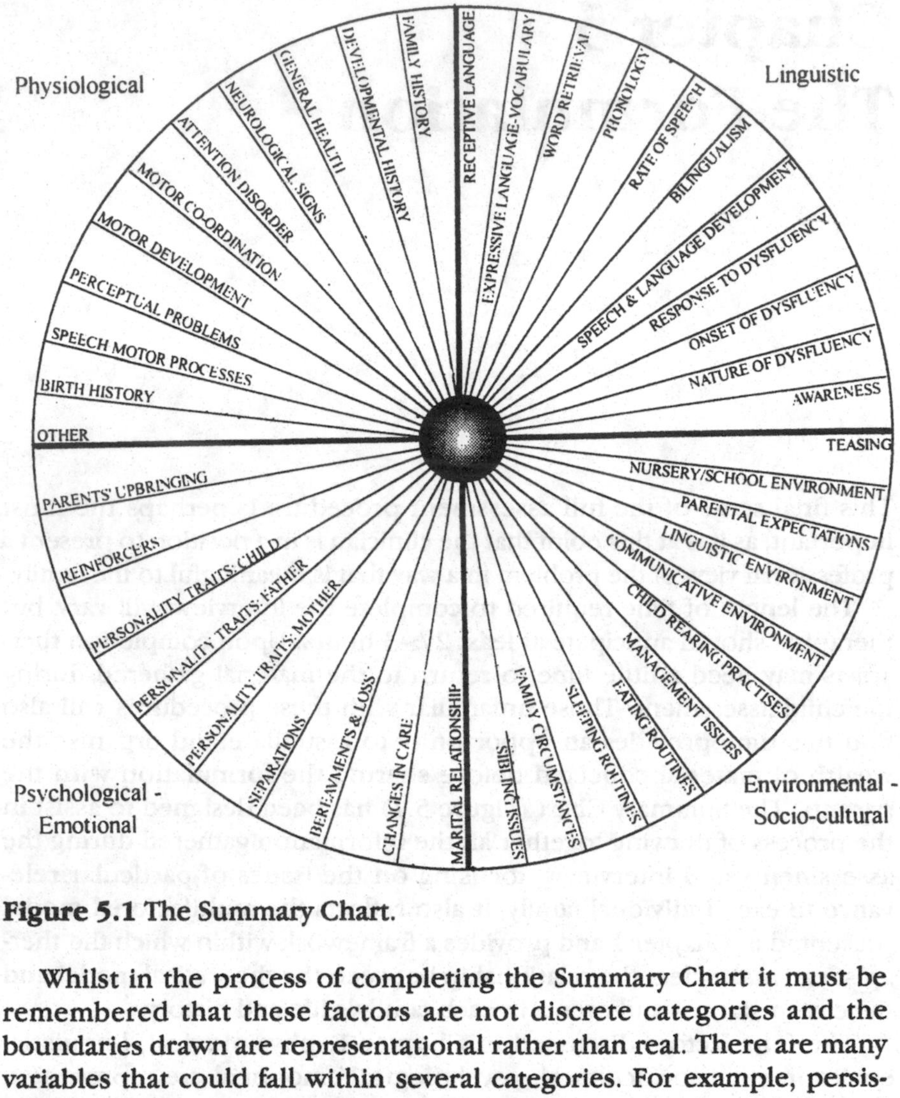

Figure 5.1 The Summary Chart.

Whilst in the process of completing the Summary Chart it must be remembered that these factors are not discrete categories and the boundaries drawn are representational rather than real. There are many variables that could fall within several categories. For example, persistent bedwetting may be seen as physiological, emotional, psychological or, indeed, as a question of management and therefore an environmental factor. The clinician will be able to decide where to place it on the Summary Chart in the light of other information gathered in the case history.

Having highlighted the areas of special relevance to a particular family, the clinician is ready to formulate an hypothesis about the nature of the child's problem and present it to the parents with recommendations for therapy. However, it is helpful if parents and therapists can share from the beginning an understanding of the nature of dysfluency and stuttering. It is important therefore to begin the formulation by informing parents of some of the generally accepted facts about dysfluency and stuttering available in the literature (see Appendix V).

We begin by restating that there is no *single* cause that can explain stuttering but it is generally accepted that there is a combination of individual factors that seem to make one person more vulnerable than another. We tell the parents that stuttering has been recorded throughout history, for example, Moses was described as being 'heavy of tongue'; Isaiah 32:4 says 'And the tongues of stutterers shall be ready to speak plainly'; Demosthenes, the Greek philosopher, was told to put pebbles in his mouth to help him become fluent. Furthermore, stuttering has been recorded in all cultures, it occurs in all socio-economic groups and within all levels of intelligence. The research indicates that there are more boys who stutter than girls, the ratio being 3:1 increasing to as much as 5 or 6:1 as they grow older with more girls seeming to 'recover' than boys.

We explain that it is, in the main, a disorder of childhood, usually occurring between the ages of 2–5 years. Approximately 5% of children will be dysfluent at some time, some of whom will recover as they pass through a temporary period of normal dysfluency. Many, however, will need help to recover their speech and 1% will continue to stutter into adult life.

The clinician continues with an explanation of the four factors on the Summary Chart. Presenting each factor in turn, the clinician may then refer to the relevant research, relating this to the appropriate information gathered from the assessments. For example, referring to research concerning the genetic predisposition where a child has a positive family history. It is important to present the research information in terms that the parents will be able to understand, avoiding jargon where possible.

Physiological factors

We tell them about the increasing evidence that the predisposition to stutter is inherited and that the child most at risk is the son of a mother who stutters, but that not all stutterers have a family history, so the genetic factor alone does not account for all stuttering (Kidd, 1977; Kidd, Kidd and Records, 1978; Andrews et al., 1983; Pauls, 1990). We then make reference to the research into the brain function of people who stutter, as there is evidence that some people who stutter use both sides of the brain for speech, whereas fluent speakers tend to use solely the left (Moore and Boberg, 1987). Similarly, it is suggested that some stutterers have difficulty retrieving, organising or sequencing the words they need to express their thoughts. Others seem to take a little longer to organise the complex and intricate movements of their tongue, lips, vocal cords and breathing for speech (Adams, Freeman and Conture, 1985; Peters and Hulstijn, 1987). Having described these aspects of the research, the clinician can then reflect back to the parents the important factors that have emerged from the assessments that are evidence of some physiological base to the child's difficulty. For example, a family history of stuttering, a clumsy child with poor motor development, a traumatic birth history, feeding difficulties, etc. would be relevant here.

Linguistic factors

The parents are informed of the research which indicates that children who have other speech and language difficulties are more at risk of fluency breakdown, a fact that is particularly relevant to this young age group which is in the process of acquiring these skills. There is also evidence that the slower a stutterer speaks the more likely they are to be fluent. This phenomenon is often intuitively understood by parents who frequently express the view that 'the child's brain is working faster than his mouth'. Sharing the results of all the assessments of the child's speech and language skills will enable the parents to understand the implications of these findings on their child's communicative difficulties, and the remediation that may be necessary in order to resolve them.

Environmental/sociocultural factors

Here we explain the implications from the research that childrens' speech and language skills are influenced by the environment within which they are developing. It is important to link those factors in the lifestyle of each child which could be increasing the risk of fluency breakdown. These may include children who are in competition with siblings, chaotic households, inconsistent management, rapid and/or complex linguistic environment, bi- or trilingual families, teasing or bullying at school, etc. Each family will present with its own unique pattern of variables and each dysfluent child will respond differently to these. As a result of the interview the therapist will have gained a picture of those factors that seem most relevant to a particular child, and should present these to the parents at this point in the formulation.

Psychological/emotional factors

At this stage it is important to dispel the myth that exists that stuttering is caused by 'nerves'. We explain to the parents that stutterers as a group are no different psychologically from a group of fluent speakers, but that motor skills can be affected by our emotional state. For example, the typist who is usually fast and accurate is more likely to make mistakes when under pressure from her boss and anxious to succeed. We explain that speech is a motor skill and is often directly affected by our emotional state. It is at this point that the therapist can relate the emotional characteristics of the child to the difficulties the child is having communicating and, where appropriate, the influence other family members' personalities have on this. For example, a child who is described as 'easy going, friendly and sociable' will be able to cope much more successfully with his dysfluency than one described as a 'worrier and a perfectionist'. A parent who shares similar characteristics will perhaps compound the situation, either positively or negatively. This is also the time to discuss important emotional issues that have been disclosed during the assessments, explaining the ways in which these may be contributing to, exacerbating or maintaining the current problem, for example, marital discord or depression. Some parents have great difficulty discussing and coping with emotional issues, a pattern which becomes repeated in their children. Recognising the effect this has on the child and the speech difficulty needs to be discussed with the parents.

As clinicians become more experienced in this procedure they will be able to identify the key issues in a family where many factors are contributing to the child's dysfluency. If all the factors are discussed at this stage parents could become overwhelmed, which would clearly be counterproductive. Selecting one or two key issues and presenting them alongside a package of remediation will direct the formulation to a positive conclusion enabling parents to leave the assessment feeling confident about the help they are to receive. Opportunities for the clinician to address the other issues identified during the assessment will become apparent during therapy and are discussed in Chapter 7.

Although clinicians will vary in the style and manner in which they feedback information to the parents, we have found it helpful to adopt an empathetic approach, identifying positive factors as well as the areas of difficulty, and pausing frequently to check the parents have understood.

Case Study

Jonathan, age: 4;4
Assessment results:

Cognitive skills:	systematic approach to formboards, using trial and error strategies appropriate play
Comprehension:	*British Picture Vocabulary Scale* Standard score 110 Age equivalent 5;0 years Responded to commands involving five information-carrying words. Evidence of superior skills
Expressive language:	Renfrew *Word Finding Vocabulary Scale* Age equivalent 5;0 years Evidence of good expressive language skills

	Evidence of slightly delayed phonological development affecting intelligibility at times
	Creaky voice quality
	Monotonous tone
Social skills:	Well developed and age-appropriate
Fluency:	3% dysfluency
	155 words spoken per minute
	Jonathan was very fluent on the assessment occasion. However, there was evidence of tense pauses and some struggle.
	Rapid rate of speech contributes to dysfluency and to poor intelligibility.

The formulation was presented to Jonathan's parents as follows:

There are four factors that seem to be important in determining if a child is at risk of developing a stutter, the first is physiological. There has been considerable research directed at trying to find a physical cause for stuttering, and it has now become clear that the predisposition to stutter may be inherited. That is, if it is in the family, it is much more likely to occur again in the same family and the person at greatest risk is the son of a mother who stutters. The fact that Jonathan's uncle and grandfather stuttered clearly puts him at risk. However, that is not enough to create the problem; as you know there are other children in the family who do not stutter. There has also been research into the brain function of stutterers, trying to find ways in which this differs from fluent speakers. There is evidence that some stutterers use both sides of their brain for speech, whereas fluent speakers commonly use the left alone. There is also evidence that stutterers as a group have difficulty with, and need more time to retrieve, organise and sequence the words they need to express their thoughts. Some also take longer to transfer these messages to the organs of articulation and have difficulty coordinating the movements necessary for fluent speech. If we look at all the information you have given me about Jonathan's physical development, although he is obviously now thriving, he did have a rather difficult start. Following his birth he had difficulties breathing and was in an incubator for a week which must have been worrying for you and although he made a good recovery, you have described him as a rather clumsy child, who finds it difficult to coordinate tasks such as doing up his buttons. He seems to have some minimal difficulties in motor coordination which are also reflected in his speech production. Again, this is not enough to create the problem but clearly could make the fine coordination of fluent speech physically more difficult for him.

Secondly, there are the linguistic factors which are important as there is considerable evidence in the research that children who have other speech and language difficulties are more vulnerable to fluency breakdown. Our assessments have shown that his understanding of spoken language is very good, he copes well with five element commands and he scored an age equivalent of 5 years on the *British Picture Vocabulary Scale*, which is a test of his understanding of spoken vocabulary, and his actual age is 4 years 4 months. His expressive language skills are also good. His vocabulary on the *Word Finding Vocabulary Scale* was also at 5.0 year level and there was no

evidence of word-finding difficulties. So, there is nothing to worry about as far as his language skills are concerned as these are above average. However, there is a considerable mismatch between this and his ability to organise the complex motor coordinations needed to express himself. He has clearly had some difficulties organising his motor processes generally and these are also reflected in the organisation of the articulators for speech. The development of his speech production was slow, immature, difficult to understand. Our brief assessment of these seems to indicate that there are, indeed, several immaturities in his system but that these seem to be resolving gradually. We also assessed Jonathan's fluency, using a tape recorded sample of his speech. There was little evidence of dysfluency on this occasion, but you say that he is in a good phase at the moment. He was dysfluent on 3% of his total speech output. However, his rate of speech was 155 words per minute where the adult norm is 120–140. This rapid rate of speech is a major contributor to his lack of intelligibility and to his dysfluency. It is also interesting to note that the dysfluency is quite tense in nature and shows clear evidence of struggle at times.

The third factor concerns the environment within which the child is developing his communication skills. There are many things that have been shown to have an influence on the development of dysfluency. It is therefore important to try to identify those that may be affecting Jonathan from all the information you have given me. The first, most important feature, being that you are obviously a very caring and supportive family unit, you (the parents) seem to have a good relationship and have worked out a lifestyle that suits you both. However, it is a very busy life that leaves little time for the maintenance of the relationship between the two of you, and it may be useful to consider setting aside some time in the week for you to spend together alone. It also seems quite difficult for Jonathan, who needs more time to do things, to compete with two very verbal, articulate sisters, in an environment that is very busy and moves at a fast pace. I have noted for instance that you, Carol, (mother) also speak at a very rapid rate and I suspect his sisters do too. Again these factors are not responsible for his dysfluency, however, given his difficulty organising the sounds for speech, they do make it much more difficult for him to have his say and be fluent. Jonathan's school has obviously been a great success but it is interesting to note that his dysfluency began at around the time he started. The increased demands of the school environment and establishing new relationships were obviously difficult for him.

The fourth and final factor is the psychological and emotional nature of the child and family. We should first dispel the myth that stuttering is caused by nerves. The research has demonstrated that stutterers are no more nervous than the rest of us. However, you have described Jonathan very clearly as a bit of a worrier, who is quite anxious about new situations and events; he doesn't like change, and likes things to be predictable. You have both been justifiably anxious about Jonathan from birth. Jonathan is quite clearly aware of his speech difficulties, he has told us so, and at times like these you both became anxious. You (mother) have also described your need to talk things through when you are worried and I think Jonathan is the same, he needs to understand and talk an issue through to lessen his anxiety. However, your experiences, John (father), during childhood of the loss of your mother and then being sent to boarding schools where you were very unhappy have taught you to bottle things up and not to discuss things of an emotional nature. Perhaps Carol and Jonathan can help and encourage you to discuss your feelings, as it will be important for Jonathan to see that this is an acceptable way of coping with difficult issues.

We can see now that there are several factors which put Jonathan at risk of stuttering, and you were right to come for help. There is an inherited predisposition, some difficulties in motor coordination generally and in the organisation of speech in particular, and it would seem that the demands he and others are placing on these skills at times outweigh his ability to deal with them and this results in dysfluency.

My recommendations for therapy therefore would be to structure some time in the week for you (the parents) to have together, maybe to go out, or simply have a drink together after the children are in bed when you can discuss the issues that have cropped up in the week. We will also arrange six weeks of interactive therapy to look at small changes you can make as a family in the way that you communicate with Jonathan that will facilitate his fluency.

Throughout this process of feedback the therapist seeks clarification from the parents that they have understood and their verbal and nonverbal reactions to what is said will indicate the accuracy of the formulations. It is often at this time that parents begin to see the complex way in which all these factors interact and understand the role they might play in therapy. Parents will often need to be reassured during this session that they have not caused the problem nor are they in some way dysfunctional families or inadequate parents. Nonetheless, an appreciation of their essential role in facilitating the child's fluency is fundamental to successful therapy.

Recommendations for therapy

In most cases this would involve six weekly sessions of 1 hour's interaction therapy, which is described in Chapter 6, but it may also include a range of other recommendations. The physiological factors may indicate a need for a further investigation of hearing, sight, general health or further psychological or neurological testing.

The linguistic factors may suggest a need for further, more in-depth speech or language evaluations, leading to remediation strategies for these specific difficulties. The environmental factors may require referral to other agencies, such as a child guidance, housing, social services, etc.

Finally, the psychological factors may indicate a need for counselling services of various kinds, for example, bereavement or marital therapy.

These recommendations can be included where appropriate, though therapists who have had further training in counselling and other related disciplines may feel able to offer these services to the family as part of their package of care.

In our clinical experience the children we have seen fall into three broad categories:

- Low risk of stuttering — minimal intervention.

- At risk of stuttering — delayed intervention.
- At risk of stuttering — intervention recommended.

Low risk of stuttering — minimal intervention

This would apply to children who are presenting with and are described as exhibiting dysfluencies which fall into the category of normal dysfluencies, who were observed to be unaware of the dysfluency, the onset of dysfluency was relatively recent (see Chapter 1) and where there are no significant features in the parent interview. Children in this group may be offered some interaction sessions to help the parents provide a communicating environment that will facilitate the child's fluency and provide an opportunity to discuss their anxieties and any other management difficulties. Continued monitoring of the family will ensure any deterioration in the dysfluency or increase in anxiety will be dealt with immediately.

At risk of stuttering — delayed intervention

Occasionally it becomes clear during the interview that whilst it is important that the family attends for therapy because the child is at risk, there are so many other areas of instability within the family that they would find it very difficult to give the time and attention necessary to therapy for a successful outcome, for example, the imminent birth of a baby, moving house, or a father's absence.

Therapists will need to be flexible according to the family's needs and circumstances.

Case Example

> Mr and Mrs T had three children: the eldest was very dysfluent which was causing great distress to the child, the parents and the family. However, at the time of interview the mother was 8 months pregnant and had to travel a considerable distance to the clinic. It was agreed to set up 'Special Times' (refer to Chapter 6 regarding Special Times) but postpone the interaction therapy until the new baby was born and the family had settled down into a new routine. The family sent in task sheets each week regarding the 'Special Times' and therapy commenced as soon as they felt ready.

At risk of stuttering — intervention recommended

Those children and families considered at risk are taken on for 6 weeks of interaction therapy. This is followed by 6 weeks' consolidation after which the therapist will reassess the position and may include (a) some sessions of direct work on the dysfluency or (b) work directly on language/phonology and sometimes both. However, it has been our experience that during the 6 weeks' consolidation many changes take place. In some cases spontaneous improvements are noted by parents and therapist in the child's language and or phonology. The interaction therapy seems to directly influence much more than fluency, it taps into language learning specifically (Kelman and Schneider, 1994; Rustin, 1995), providing the optimum environment for the development of speech and language skills. We have also found that parents, encouraged and empowered by their success in making changes in their interactions with the dysfluent child, begin to make small changes in other areas of family life. For example, restructuring bedtimes so that younger children go to bed in advance of their elders. It is also significant that once these changes have been made and the children have become more fluent, those that do need direct intervention only require minimal help. The levels of fluency gained by individual children will vary, however it is the parents' confidence in their ability to manage the child's dysfluency that seems more important at this stage. Parents report that these children acquire skills and incorporate them into their repertoire quickly and easily, in the same way that they might learn to use a knife and fork rather than a spoon once one has been proved more effective than the other.

Most of the children we see in our clinic are tertiary referrals or children who have waited for several months without therapy with no spontaneous improvement, thus most fall into the third category. Whatever the circumstances, however, this form of therapy is short, relatively cost-effective, efficacious, and may prevent the development of a long term problem.

The following cases illustrate the formulation procedure we have described in this chapter. They are a representative sample demonstrating the different combination of factors that emerge as significant for each child. In these examples we have described the main features of the parental interview and the child assessment and identified the key factors on a Summary Chart.

Case Study

George, age: 3;2
Assessment results:

Cognitive skills:	Organisational skills good for simple tasks, but few problem-solving skills on more complex tasks Right handed Play: appropriate
Comprehension:	*British Picture Vocabulary Scale* Standard score 97 Age equivalent 2;10 Responded to commands involving three information-carrying words Syntax and Semantics: age-appropriate
Expressive language:	Renfrew *Word Finding Vocabulary Scale* Age equivalent 3;0

	Using simple structures
	Wide vocabulary
	No evidence of word-finding difficulties
	Phonology immature at times
	Unintelligible in discourse
Social skills:	Good
Fluency:	2.9 % dysfluency
	117 words spoken per minute
	George was very fluent on the assessment occasion, there was evidence of part-word and whole-word repetitions on initiation and interruptions.
	There was no evidence of awareness.

George was aged 3;2 months when his family attended for assessment. His mother, Lucy, had referred him, somewhat ambivalently, as she had been hoping he would outgrow the problem. However, his repetitive speech pattern and initiation problems had become noticeable to others, and Lucy was concerned that he might be teased.

Lucy and George's father, Carl, attended the parent interview. They described George's rather complex medical history. Whilst Lucy was pregnant with him she suffered viral meningitis and at 26 weeks she was given antibiotics intravenously. George was born at 42 weeks with the umbilical cord around his neck, and was resuscitated. He had a heart murmur and a congenital hip deformity. At 3 weeks he developed severe eczema with open sores which was subsequently controlled through his diet. He was put into a parachute harness for his hip from 6 weeks until 7 months. When he was 2½ years old he developed asthma which was treated with a nebuliser three times per day. His heart murmur was being monitored and it was expected that he would require surgery for a fistula at around 10 years. In spite of these medical problems George's general health was good, he had no hearing or sight problems, a healthy appetite and slept well.

George's developmental milestones were normal apart from delayed phonological development which made him unintelligible to all except his immediate family, causing George to become frustrated and aggressive at times. His dysfluency had emerged gradually from 12 months when he began to talk. This coincided with the birth of his sister as well as his mother's hospitalisation for one week with a pulmonary embolus, during which time George stayed with his grandparents.

George had an older brother of 4 years who was inclined to dominate him and a younger sister of 2 years who was bright and verbal. They all played, squabbled and fought together. Lucy and Carl tried to give each child individual time but this frequently proved impossible and the children often showed jealousy of each other. George also had a cousin of the same age who was bossy and articulate. The family had a busy social life and was very involved with extended family members, in daily contact and sharing holidays together.

Lucy and Carl described their own relationship as being fine, they enjoyed each other's company as well as their social life with friends. Carl had recently been made redundant from his job as a car dealer and was running a market stall at weekends. Lucy worked part time as a dental hygienist. They said their financial status was 'worrying' but their lifestyle was stable. Lucy described her personality as bossy, independent, assertive and capable; Carl described himself as shy, lacking in confidence and untidy. Neither parent suffered any health problems and there was no family history of stuttering. Both parents reported that they had a happy stable upbringing.

Table 5.1 Issues for George

Physiological	*Linguistic*
Birth: asphyxia Eczema/asthma Heart defect	Phonology
Psychological/emotional	*Environmental/sociocultural*
Separation from mother at 12 months Frustration, aggression Parents anxious re money and George's health	Sibling rivalry Turn-taking Social life Hectic lifestyle

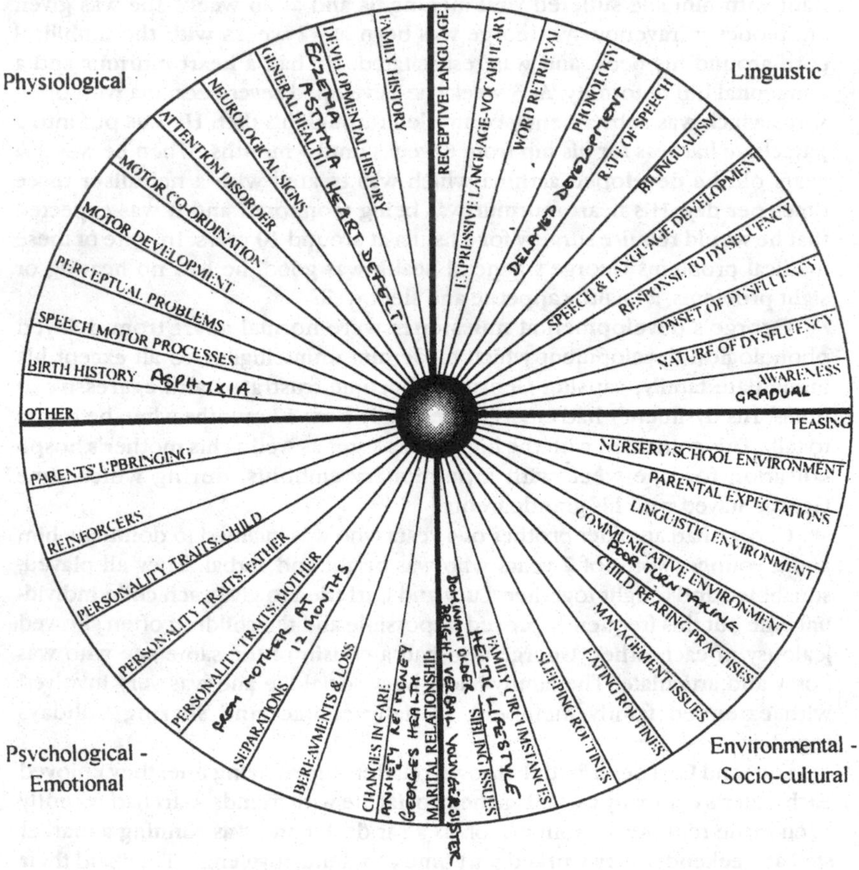

Figure 5.2 Summary Chart: George, age 3;2.

Case Study

Chris, age: 5;4
Assessment results:

Cognitive skills:	**Organised, logical and confident approach to form-boards and abacus, appropriate play**
Comprehension:	***British Picture Vocabulary Scale***
	Standard score: 96
	Age equivalent: 4;11
	Responded to commands involving five information-carrying words
	Some syntactic immaturities
Expressive language:	**Renfrew *Word Finding Vocabulary Scale***
	Age equivalent: 5 years
	Some naming difficulties when no picture cues, benefit from additional time to formulate language
	Evidence of specific word-finding difficulties
	Some phonological immaturities
Social skills:	**Appropriate except limited eye contact during dysfluency**
Fluency:	**32.9 percentage dysfluency**
	49 words spoken per minute
	whole-word and part-word repetitions; prolongations and struggle behaviour, hand movements, disrupted breathing pattern
	Some evidence of awareness

Chris was aged 5;4 when we assessed him, he was the only child of a single mother who lived with her own mother and two foster sisters, 14 and 17 years old. Chris had only limited contact with his father because he was not welcomed by the other members of the family. The interview and assessments demonstrated clearly that Chris was at risk of stuttering. Chris's general health was poor he had persistent bouts of vomiting, headache and drowsiness which had not yet been adequately explained or treated by his GP. He was described by his mother as being rather clumsy and poorly coordinated with a short concentration span. There was a family history of stuttering as Chris' uncle (mother's brother) stuttered as a child. There was a reported delay in the development of receptive and expressive language which was supported by the assessments Chris completed during the child assessment. The *British Picture Vocabulary Scale* score gave an age-equivalent of 4;11. The *Word Finding Vocabulary Scale* indicated specific word-finding difficulties and use of gesture. The dysfluency was persistent with no periods of fluency reported. The fluency assessment indicated that Chris stuttered 32.9% of his total output and he spoke at a rate of 49 words per minute. There was evidence of part-word repetitions, prolongations and struggle behaviour which was characterised by changes in volume and pitch, disrupted breathing and observable tension around the mouth. Concomitant movements were noted during moments of struggle, both hands raised and sometimes he slapped his knee.

The sample of Chris's discourse clearly demonstrated an increase in dysfluency as the demand on his linguistic skills increased, unstructured discourse being the most dysfluent. The speech sample also demonstrated Chris's phonological difficulties which contributed to his poor intelligibility. There was clear evidence that Chris's speech and language difficulties were closely related to his dysfluency.

The linguistic environment also presented some problems for Chris. His mother spoke very rapidly and the predominantly adult models of language available at home suggest a level of linguistic complexity beyond Chris's abilities. His mother was very caring and concerned to do her best for him, and there were few significant features amongst the emotional factors. However, the difficult relationship between Chris's mother and his father, and the uncertain nature of *his* relationship with his father were clearly important. Chris and his mother were hoping to be moved to their own accommodation within the next few months which would effect a major change in their lifestyle and would require careful management.

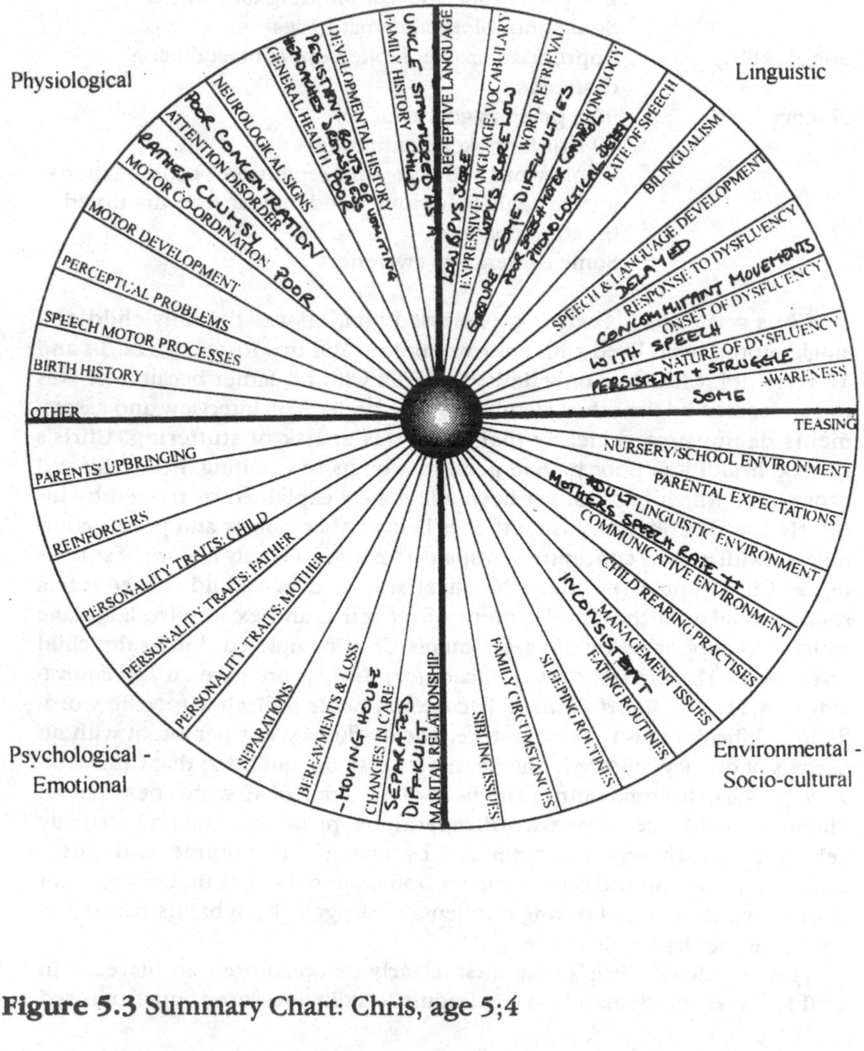

Figure 5.3 Summary Chart: Chris, age 5;4

Table 5.2 Issues for Chris

Physiological	*Linguistic*
Family history	BPVS score low
Poor concentration	WPVS score low
Poor coordination	Delayed speech and language milestones
	Speech motor control phonology
	Onset with speech *no* periods of fluency
	Evidence of struggle and concomitant movements
Psychological/emotional	***Environmental/sociocultural***
Relationship with father	Mother's speech rate
Moving house to place on own	Management inconsistent
	Complexity of adult language model

Case Study

Catherine, age: 4;7

Assessment results:

Cognitive skills:	Good organisational skills
	Hand preference not firmly established
	Imaginative play
Comprehension:	*British Picture Vocabulary Scale*
	Standard score: 105
	Age equivalent: 4;9
	Responding to commands involving five information-carrying words
Expressive language:	Renfrew *Word Finding Vocabulary Scale*
	Age equivalent: 4;4
	Evidence of simple and complex sentence structures
	Some evidence of word retrieval difficulties
	Phonology age-appropriate
Social skills:	Generally immature
	Listening and attention skills poor
	Poor turn-taking, frequent interruptions
	Poor eye contact
	Frequently seeking adult attention
Fluency:	7.9% dysfluency
	133 words spoken per minute
	Whole-word repetitions up to 3
	Prolongations 1–2 seconds
	Struggle evident
	Creaky voice quality
	Evidence of word avoidance and awareness of difficulty
	Hand movements, disrupted breathing pattern
	Some evidence of awareness

David and Janet had three children: Jane, Catherine and Sarah. Catherine was 3 when she became very dysfluent after her first few days at nursery school. The onset was sudden and quite severe in nature with blocking, prolongations and facial grimacing. Since then the dysfluency had fluctuated with periods of fluency extending to several weeks. Janet had a miscarriage between Jane and Catherine, she had been very distressed and took several months to recover. The pregnancy with Catherine was difficult, ultimately requiring Janet to spend several weeks in hospital on bed rest. However, despite this, Catherine's birth was uneventful and there were no significant physiological factors reported, and no family history of stuttering.

Assessments of Catherine's speech revealed age-appropriate skills on all tests. However, the *Word Finding Vocabulary Scale* suggested some word retrieval difficulties which were also noted during the analysis of the speech sample.

The family was very warm, loving and supportive of each other. However, there was considerable competition for verbal space, both sisters were garrulous and articulate and Janet spoke very rapidly. David and Janet had a good relationship but the demands of the children and David's job made it difficult to organise time for each other.

Since the onset of the dysfluency Janet's management of Catherine's behaviour had become inconsistent with that of the rest of the family, as she was fearful of worsening the dysfluency, Catherine was allowed to 'get away with murder'.

Catherine was described as a child who was anxious to please and a worrier, just like her mother. Janet liked to have things in order and was a bit of a perfectionist. David was the calming influence, easygoing and phlegmatic, he was also a very hard worker and saw little of the family during the week. David had a comfortable stable childhood, whereas Janet had a difficult relationship with her own mother, and had a very unhappy school life.

Table 5.3 Issues for Catherine

Physiological	*Linguistic*
Difficult pregnancy	Some word retrieval Sudden onset Very aware of dysfluency Struggle behaviour Avoidance Rapid rate
Psychological/emotional	*Environmental/sociocultural*
Father: easygoing, but hard worker Mother: worrier, perfectionist Child: worrier, anxious to please Mother's relationship with own mother Mother's experiences at school	Sibling rivalry Competition for verbal space High parental expectations

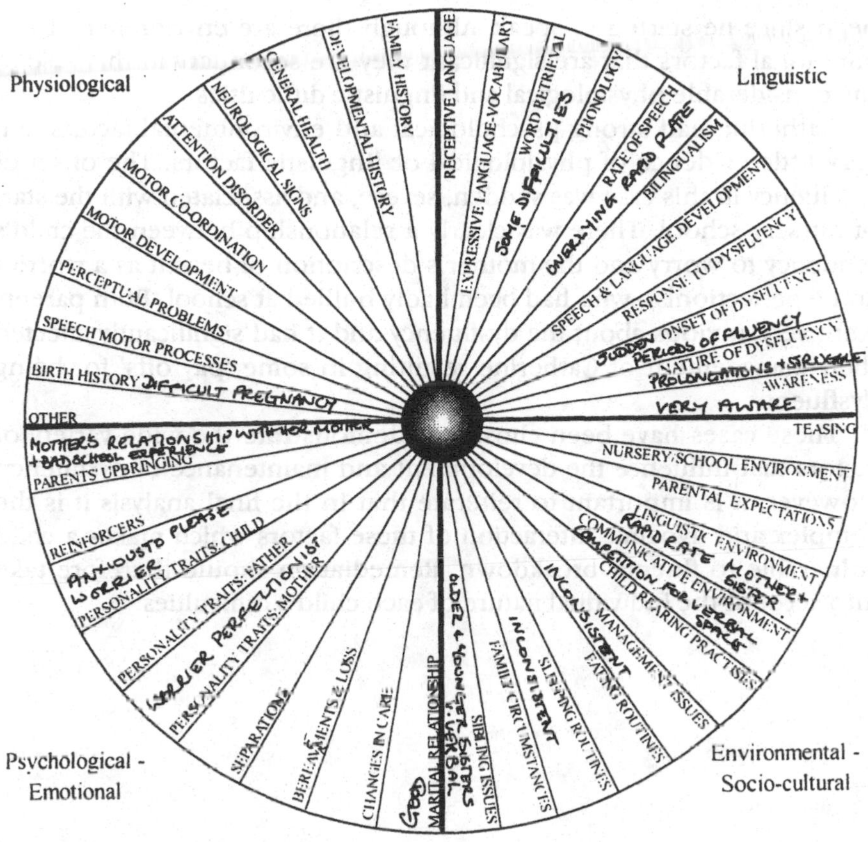

Figure 5.4 Summary Chart: Catherine, aged 3;6

These case histories demonstrate the wide range of issues that present in the clinic. Understanding the individual nature of each child's difficulties and the unique combination of physiological, linguistic, environmental and emotional factors enables the clinician to explain to the parents why this child is vulnerable to fluency breakdown and describe remediation that will address the problem.

George presented a case which had a strong physiological base though no family history. There was evidence of speech motor control difficulties from very early on in George's development. This was then compounded by a number of emotional and environmental variables, such as the separation from his mother at 12 months, the birth of his sister, sibling rivalry and a busy and sometimes chaotic lifestyle.

Chris's study described a 3-year-old boy with a strong physiological and linguistic base to his dysfluency. His uncle stuttered and he had a long history of speech and language difficulties associated with poor coordination and speech motor control. Chris's dysfluency was persistent and had been since he started to speak. Although there are environmental and emotional factors that are significant they are secondary in this case to the considerable physiological and linguistic difficulties.

Catherine had strong psychological and environmental factors and very little evidence of physiological or linguistic factors. The onset of dysfluency in this case was sudden, severe, and associated with the start of nursery school. There was clearly a relationship between the child's tendency to worry and the mother's description of herself as a worrier and a perfectionist, who had been badly bullied at school. Both parents were very anxious about the dysfluency and it had significantly affected their management of Catherine resulting in some 'pay offs' for being dysfluent.

These cases have been chosen to demonstrate the wide variety of factors that influence the development and maintenance of dysfluency. However, it is important to reiterate that in the final analysis it is the complex and dynamic interaction of these factors which makes a child vulnerable to fluency breakdown. Remediation should therefore take into account the individual nature of each child's difficulties.

Chapter 6
Interaction Therapy

Introduction

During the assessment, parents frequently report their distress and feelings of helplessness when faced with their child's dysfluency. They often have little understanding of the nature of the problem, or its perplexing variability and are unable to predict what will exacerbate or remediate it. They feel disempowered by this experience and often begin to abandon their normal parenting practices in an attempt to bring the dysfluency under control. The principal aim of this therapeutic approach is to help parents restore their confidence in their parenting skills, to understand the complexity of this disorder and to find ways of interacting with the child that will facilitate fluency.

Interaction therapy enables parents to observe their own communicative style, and encourages them to become objective in their evaluations of their own behaviour. This process helps parents discover the many positive as well as negative effects of their interactional style, and enables them to make the small self-determined changes which are the cornerstone of this therapy. Developing the parents' skills in this way allows them to take control of the problem as they assist their child in ways that *they* can understand, regulate and monitor.

Structure of therapy

A contract is made with both the parents for a fixed-term treatment period of six weeks. Once-weekly appointments lasting an hour should be arranged. The weekly interval is necessary to facilitate home practice of new skills learned in the clinic setting. Following the six treatment sessions, there is a review period when the changed styles of interaction are consolidated. It is during this period that the effects of interaction therapy on the child's fluency should become apparent. The family is seen again to monitor the parents' and child's progress at the end of the consolidation period when decisions are made as to further input.

Both parents participate in all stages of interaction therapy, and other caregivers should be involved as necessary. This could involve nannies or au pairs who are responsible for the child's day-to-day management as well as grandparents, siblings, etc.

Where couples are separated, therapy sessions should be arranged for each parent and the child individually.

First therapy session

The first therapy session begins with the setting of the 'Special Time' task. This is a modification of the Talking Time task described in the *Assessment and Therapy Programme for Dysfluent Children* (Rustin, 1987).

'Special Time' task

The purpose of the task is as follows:

- It gives an indication of the parents' commitment to therapy.
- It provides the child with quality time with each parent which is beneficial in its own right.
- It provides a structure in which the parents can practise target behaviours, which are to be identified in future weeks.

Both parents are given a copy of the Special Time instruction sheet (see Figure 6.1). Each parent is asked to decide how frequently they could undertake the task in a week, with a minimum of three times and a maximum of six times per week. Realistic targets should be encouraged as it is important for parents to be able to succeed in this task. Parents may insist that they want to do the task on a daily basis, however, we would encourage them to lower their targets initially and then increase the number if it is going well. Some discussion may be necessary if a parent's contact with the child is limited, e.g. working parents might find that early in the morning before they leave is the best time.

When the parents have read the instruction sheet various points are reiterated:

- The Special Time must be restricted to 5 minutes: parents often want to extend the time, especially if the child protests that he wants to continue. It is explained that the time limit is essential to the success of the Special Time because it means the task is achievable even in a busy lifestyle. It is also a realistic time slot for practising and maintaining changes in styles of interaction. It is important that the parents establish and adhere to the strict timing in the first week

SPECIAL TIME - INSTRUCTION SHEET

Special Time lasts for five minutes only and should not be extended.

Allow your child to select an activity, toy or game of his choice. This should not be reading a book, watching television or playing a lively outdoor game. When the child has chosen what to do, go to a room where you will not be disturbed and deal with any obvious distractions eg T.V., radio. Play with your child, focusing your attention on him/her and what he or she is saying (not how he or she is saying it). When the allotted time has finished record your Special Time on the task sheet, writing what you did and how you felt about it.

Figure 6.1 Special Time instruction sheet.

of therapy, in order that the child understands that the Special Time is limited. Parents often find it useful to use an egg timer to allow the child to monitor the 5 minutes and recognise when it has come to an end.

- The Special Time is not to be used as an opportunity to observe and record the child's fluency levels. Parents may misinterpret the purpose of the task and focus on *how* the child is speaking instead of on *what* he is saying.

The parents are then given task sheets to complete (see Appendix VII) describing the play activity as well as their own reaction to the Special Time. Examples of comments may be given, e.g. *'It was fun' 'I really enjoyed playing with Tom'* or *'I didn't realise he has such a good imagination' 'I was tired today and didn't feel like playing'*.

The remainder of the first session should be used to discuss any queries arising from the summary of the assessment findings and the formulation. It is important to remember that parents will not have retained all the information given to them at the end of the parent interview. They should be encouraged to ask questions or feedback their reaction to the summary, having had time to reflect upon it and discuss it together. This session enhances the clinician–parent relationship contributing to the development of trust and establishing a working partnership.

Session format

The subsequent sessions follow a seven-point format:

1. Review of 'Special Times', including collection of task sheets.
2. Video recording of each parent playing individually with their child.
3. Parents and clinician view video and identify target behaviours to change.
4. Video recording of parents playing individually with their child implementing targeted change.
5. Parents and clinician view second video to discuss progress.
6. Targeted change to be practised in Special Times at home and recorded on task sheets.
7. Discussion of specific issues within the family.

Review of 'Special Times'

The clinician reads the task sheets and then discusses with both parents any issues relating to their homework task. We are interested in whether they have achieved their target number of Special Times, so fulfilling their commitment to the task. If a parent has done fewer Special Times than they elected to do, the reasons for this should be explored. Since the task is a measure of commitment to therapy as a whole, it would be inappropriate to proceed with the treatment programme if a parent has failed at this stage. The task would need to be discussed again and the parents invited to review the target number of 'Special Times'. They are then instructed to carry out the task for another week before interaction therapy can begin.

Parents sometimes complete the task but have extended the time, especially where children have protested at the end of 5 minutes. If this becomes the expected pattern parents may find themselves unable to set aside enough time. It is therefore essential to establish, for all concerned, that 5 minutes is sufficient to complete the task. Problems of this nature can be discussed with the parents and the task re-set. It is important that interaction therapy is not commenced until the 'Special Time' task is completed.

Case Example

Jason, aged 3;2, attended with his parents, Michael and Janine. Michael worked long hours as a systems analyst sometimes on night or weekend shifts. Janine was at home with their three children: Jason, John aged 5, and Ryan, aged 11 months. At the beginning of therapy Michael agreed to a commitment of four Special Times per week and Janine said she would do five. After one week the parents reported back their tasks. Michael had done four special times with Jason, completing his task sheet. He commented on one occasion that Jason had chosen to play with the Playmobil helicopter. This had taken almost 5 minutes to assemble so Michael extended the special time for a further 5 minutes to allow for playing. This was discussed and it was explained that extending the time was unhelpful in the long term. The previously listed reasons were reiterated and the task reset. Janine had completed three of her five Special Times, finding it very difficult to spend time with Jason on his own. Practical arrangements were discussed and it was agreed that the target be reduced to three, two of these being at the weekend when Michael was usually available to look after the other children, and one special time to be undertaken during the week. The parents were given another set of task sheets to complete by the following session. On their return a week later both parents reported that their tasks had been successfully completed. Interaction therapy then commenced.

We are also interested in the parents' description of the activity they were engaged in with the child during the Special Time as it allows the clinician to ensure that these continue to be child-directed and provide a suitable environment for successful interaction. For example, parents may record the activity as playing 'I spy' in the car on the way to school. This situation is not appropriate as the parent is unable to give their undivided attention and interaction is limited by the circumstances. The comments section on the homework sheet will also provide further information that therapists may find helpful. For example, the parents' comments may become directed towards the child's level of dysfluency; we have found that encouraging parents to make comments on their own feelings about the interaction or other aspects of the communication promotes an important shift of focus, away from the child's speech production.

First video recording

Each parent is asked to play with the child individually whilst being video-recorded. The play session should be similar to the 'Special Time', i.e. the child selects the activity and the parent and child play for 5 minutes. The video may be made by use of either a remote-controlled camera or a portable system.

Video viewing to target changes

The parents then watch this video recordings with the clinician and each parent is his or her asked to comment on aspects of their own video recording as described below. It is important to note that parents are discouraged from commenting on each other's performance. We are aiming to develop parents' self-monitoring skills and this should not evolve into a situation where the parents criticise each other. The clinician goes through this stage with each parent individually (the other parent being present but not invited to comment). The child is also in the room and may watch the videos with the parents or play on his own:

- How did the parents feel during the play session? Were they self-conscious, ill at ease, or oblivious of the camera. It is reassuring for a nervous parent to be given permission to acknowledge feelings of unease or embarrassment.
- Whether the parents' behaviour on the video is typical of a normal play session with their child. This gives the parents an opportunity to explain if they feel that the video recording is not a true representation of their usual interaction style. If the parents state that it is not typical they are encouraged to specify how their behaviour is different. It is interesting to note that many parents who were very uneasy about the camera actually reported that their play with the child was largely unaffected.
- The parents identify at least one positive feature of their behaviour. The purpose of this task is to develop parents' self-observation and monitoring skills — objectively identifying factors which may be influencing their child. It is important to focus in the first instance on a positive feature. Parents need reinforcement and reassurance that they are able to interact helpfully with their child. Parents may find this task rather embarrassing or difficult and often attempt to focus on something negative, but it is important to stop them at this point, reiterate the instruction and encourage them to be positive about themselves.
- The therapist reinforces this, adding any other positive features noted, that the parents may have overlooked. The parents then identify one aspect of their interaction which may not be so helpful. It is important to point out to the parents that it is not their communicative styles that are in question, but the effect that these have on a child's fluency. A parent may be using the same style with their other children, with no detrimental effects. This is a critical stage in the process of helping the parents develop an awareness of how they may be able to assist their child in becoming more fluent. We feel it is essential to encourage parents to develop these skills and make small changes in their behaviour based on viewing videos of themselves. In this way they are able to take ownership of the improvements in the child's fluency.

Many parents have no difficulty in identifying a relevant feature for change, for example:

- *'I don't stop asking questions and I'm not even waiting for the answers.'*

- *'I'm so bossy.'*
- *'I never realised I spoke so quickly, I can't even understand what I'm saying.'*

However, if the parents are unable to do this they may be assisted by some cueing from the clinician who might ask, *'Who is doing all the talking?' 'What about questions?' 'Tell me about your rate/speed of talking'*. If parents still find it difficult to identify factors, we give them a simple checklist of behaviours (Table 6.1), which they can use to help evaluate themselves.

Table 6.1 Checklist of behaviours for parents

Who is in charge?
Who is doing most of the talking?
Who is listening?
Who is looking?
Who is interrupting?
Who is asking questions?
How fast are we speaking?

We ask the parents to select from the checklist one item which is relevant to their behaviour. Once the parent has identified the specific behaviour, the clinician and parents explore why this particular feature is relevant to the child's fluency, e.g. *'You have noticed that you are in charge of play, telling your child what to do and not really going along with what he seems to want to do. How do you think this might have some impact on his fluency? ... It is possible that your choice of activity could be different to what your child wants to do, and it may be more sophisticated or complicated. This means your child is having to operate at a higher level, both in play and verbally, than he would naturally. He is therefore under pressure during the play and this pressure might be affecting his fluency. We need to take away as many pressures as we can, so how could we change this?'*

Having discussed various strategies, it is important to ensure that the parents are clear as to the nature of the change to be attempted and *how* this might be carried out, for instance: *'Let's try it again but this time let him take the lead in play and you follow his cue. Watch him and listen to him and join in with his play, but try not to take over.'*

Further examples of other therapy techniques are presented at the end of this chapter. This process of identifying an unhelpful aspect of the parents' behaviour for change may lead to increased feelings of guilt or a sense of having caused the child's dysfluency. It is important at this stage to reiterate that parents are not responsible for stuttering and to explain the bidirectional influences in parent–child interaction. For example, if a child is quiet and passive this forces parents into a more directive and verbal style; the behaviour of the parent is affected by the child, just as the child's behaviour is affected by the parent.

Second video recording

Having identified the change that is to be implemented the parents are once more video-recorded playing with their child individually. During this second play session each parent attempts to make the targeted change in their interaction with the child. Some parents find this difficult and it is therefore important to allow ample time so that the therapist can shape, encourage and guide the parents towards their goal. When the parents have successfully changed their behaviour for a segment of the recording, the play session is stopped in order to watch the video again. It is extremely rare for parents to be unable to implement the targeted change if they have fully understood it and discussed how they will implement it. If they do fail it is important to identify the reasons why. If they have not understood how they are to change it may be helpful for the clinician to demonstrate the change in a role play of the activity. Alternatively, the clinician may model the behaviour whilst playing with the child. We are concerned, however, that modelling might be deskilling for a parent, in that a child might respond in the required way to the clinician whom he does not know well, then revert to his usual pattern with the parents, so it should be used only if other methods fail.

Video viewing to review progress

The clinician and both parents then view the second video recording in order to provide feedback on whether the targeted change has been implemented. It is important to encourage the parents to observe their own behaviour in order to develop self-monitoring skills. Firstly, identify at least one positive feature, for example, any attempts to make the changes, even if their efforts are not entirely successful. Secondly, parents are invited to describe the experience of changing their interactive style, for instance, the feelings of self-consciousness, or lack of spontaneity. They may also be encouraged to observe any consequent changes in the child's behaviour, for example, if a parent is being less directive, does the child become a more active and verbal participant in the interaction? The clinician should also provide positive reinforcement for the parents, encouraging them to persist by rewarding the smallest of changes in the desired direction.

Home practice

The parents are instructed to implement the targeted change within their Special Times at home, for example, attempt to slow their speech rate during the 5 minutes' play with their child. At this point, we emphasise the importance of the parents using the Special Time for practice, but not attempting to change their behaviour the rest of the time. We aim to prevent the parents from being too ambitious and failing. Making changes at all times would not be possible and parents need to appreciate this for themselves and their child. Smaller, realistic goals encourage them in their progress; regular practice of the change will help to make it more natural and spontaneous, facilitating automatic transfer to daily life. The parents are each given a new task sheet and instructed to record on this whether they made the change and how they felt, as well as any observations of changes in the child.

It should be mentioned here that the target change may remain the same for several sessions until such time as the parents and clinician feel it has been integrated into the parents' interactive style and we would caution clinicians against moving too quickly in interaction therapy. Introducing a new behaviour change can often disrupt a previously learned skill, for instance, if parents have succeeded in slowing their rate one week and then focuses on reducing questions the next, they may find their rate increasing again as they attempt to reduce the number of questions. Under there circumstances it may be helpful to continue practising these two skills until they are firmly established before adding a third.

Discussion of specific family issues

Each therapy session should include a period of time for the family and clinician to discuss any specific matters arising from the parent interview. However, it has been our experience that issues identified during the parent interview frequently resolve without direct intervention.

Case Example

David and Jennifer had two children, Kate 5 years, and 3½-year-old Stephen who was dysfluent. During the interview they described their difficulty getting the children settled in the evenings. Stephen and Kate went to bed at the same time as it was considered easier. However, it often took longer than they anticipated so Stephen was not asleep until 8.30 pm. The children rose early and both David and Jennifer agreed that Stephen was getting less sleep than they felt he needed, and they had noticed a relationship between Stephen's dysfluency and tiredness. During the formulation the management of bedtimes was raised and the possible benefits of staggering the bedtimes was discussed. When the clinician returned to this issue during one of the interaction sessions the parents reported that as a result of the formulation they had decided to restructure bedtimes and establish a routine. Stephen was, as a result, in bed three-quarters of an hour before Kate, they felt he was less tired and that Kate was enjoying the time she had with them on her own. Jennifer was also able to report that Kate had become easier to manage and that there had been a reduction in the bickering between the two children.

The clinician was then able to reinforce and support the parents in their efforts to maintain these new behaviours.

Further discussion about management of the most commonly occurring family issues will be found in Chapter 7.

This format is used to structure each of the six agreed sessions during the fixed-term treatment period. It is a dynamic process and the changes that occur during this time are sometimes considerable, and demonstrated each week by the parents during the video interaction session. Furthermore, change rarely occurs in isolation, so that altering one specific feature of interaction will have an effect on others. For example, a mother observed that she had taken over the play session from the child and decided that she would try to follow the child's lead. After a week of experimenting with this at home during Special Times, she returned and the video recording made on her subsequent visit demonstrated several changes:

- She had been able to follow the child's leads.
- She had reduced the amount and the complexity of her verbal contributions.
- There was an increase in pausing.
- The pace of the interaction was slower and calmer.
- There was an increase in eye contact.
- There was a change in affect evident particularly in the facial expression and warmth demonstrated by both parties.

Although not all parents will make such a wide range of changes in one session it is in this way that an apparently long list of features identified during assessment may be reduced to three or four key features targeted during the 6-week period. At the end of the final session, the consolidation period of 6 weeks is discussed and a review appointment is arranged.

Consolidation period

The Consolidation Period lasts 6 weeks and it is during this time that the skills and changes which have been identified, learned and practised during the treatment programme are assimilated into the family's daily lifestyle. The parents are instructed to undertake the Special Times on the same basis as they have been doing during the treatment period, and to record the tasks on the task sheets which they will then send to the clinician at the end of each week. The clinician should monitor these task sheets giving positive reinforcement and re-instructing as appropriate by telephone or in writing. Most parents, at some point during interaction therapy, will become aware that the changes they are making in their interactions with the child can be linked with a decrease in the child's dysfluency. This is an important discovery for parents to make as it provides proof of their ability to respond to the stutter in an effective way. However, if for any reason the fluency should deteriorate during the Consolidation Period we ask the parents to contact us immediately by telephone. They are then instructed to make a diary of the events and circumstances surrounding the breakdown in the child's fluency and are asked to contact the clinician a week later to report progress. If the deterioration in fluency persists, we invite both parents to attend with their child in order to explore possible reasons for the relapse. It is particularly important that the therapist finds out whether there are any changes occurring within the family. This could simply be illness of the child or someone within the family, a holiday, or a more serious family trauma or death, etc. In our experience parents may often report that nothing has changed and that there are no unusual circumstances. Further questioning is often necessary to identify factors which the parents may not have considered relevant or significant. It may be that the parent has had an upsetting experience which they do not think has affected the child. However, the child may instinctively have realised something was wrong and become anxious, with a subsequent deterioration in fluency. We have noticed that sometimes when a child has reached an acceptable level of fluency the parents cease their commitment to the Special Times, or revert to old patterns. In most cases a review session, discussing difficulties and re-establishing the features of interaction therapy may be all that is required.

Review

At the end of the Consolidation Period a session is arranged when the child's progress can be evaluated and the parents and clinician can decide on appropriate future action.

If the child's fluency continues to be satisfactory we would arrange a further review appointment to monitor progress in 3 months' time. It is essential that the Special Time task is maintained for at least 6 months, many parents have continued for a 2-year period and some have integrated it into their family life as a permanent feature.

If the child's fluency is still causing concern it may be appropriate to undertake direct therapy with the child, as described in Chapter 8.

Examples of interaction therapy techniques

Reducing parental directiveness

Relevance to child's fluency

If the parent is in charge of the activity it is more likely to be at a sophisticated level, putting the child under pressure to perform in a more complex way, thus placing demands on fluency. Furthermore, the parent who is controlling and directing the play is not encouraging the child's creativity and imaginative development.

Techniques to achieve change

Helping parents to observe the child's play and initially, simply imitate their actions. When they are able to do this successfully a discussion about the advantages of making one or two comments on the play is conducted and then attempted. The parent is encouraged to follow the child's lead in play, which may involve watching and waiting. If the child has become accustomed to the parent being directive, it may be some time before the child begins to take the lead.

Gaining the child's attention

Here, the parents and child may each be involved in their own activity *or* the child may be totally engrossed in what he is doing *or* the child may be highly distractible and flit from one activity to the next.

Relevance to child's fluency

If we are attempting to improve the child's fluency through changing the parent style it is fundamental that the child is attending to the parent and that the parent is successfully engaging the child during play.

Techniques to achieve change

The parents are encouraged to think of strategies which will capture the child's attention, for example:

- Touch the child or call his name then wait until the child looks up before saying any more.
- Use mystery, surprise or humour to engage the child.
- Ensure the parent's face is at the same level as the child's and check the parent is looking at the child.
- Exaggerate facial expression and become more animated.
- Hold play material at the parent's face level whenever possible to encourage the child to look at the parent.

It may be necessary to use more than one of the above strategies to engage the child and maintain attention.

Rate reduction and increased pausing

This relates to parents who speak very rapidly, rarely pause and leave scant time for the child to respond to a request or comment.

Relevance to child's fluency

Research has shown that the faster a stutterer tries to speak, the more dysfluent he becomes. A slower speaking rate allows more time to organise the various functions required for fluent speech. Furthermore, it is evident that parents who speak rapidly put their children under pressure to do the same. It is therefore essential for such parents to slow down in order to maximise the child's opportunity to be fluent.

Techniques to achieve change

The clinician models an appropriate target rate with greater pausing. The parent imitates this slower style, counting to two before responding to a child's utterance. Where the child is already speaking at a much slower rate than the parent, the parent should be encouaged to listen carefully to the child and attempt a rate similar to or just below the child's, since it is the discrepancy between the two rates that is more important than the actual rate. The parents are warned that a slower rate of speaking will feel unnatural to them. However, when they watch themselves on the subsequent video recording they discover that their speech sounds normal. Parents are encouraged to note the improved intelligibility which often accompanies a reduction in their speech rate.

Increasing physical involvement in play

Some parents adopt the 'observer' role during play — they may be watching carefully and become verbally involved, but they fail to join in with the play.

Relevance to child's fluency

It is necessary for the parents to interact with the child both physically and verbally in order for changes in the parents' style to affect the child's fluency.

Techniques to achieve change

Encourage the parents to actually play with the child like a playmate of the child's own age. If the parents are unfamiliar with how a child might play they could observe their own children playing with each other or with their peers. The parents may find it helpful to imitate the child's play, follow his lead, avoid using the play session for teaching, and have fun. Sitting or lying on the floor is more playful than using a table and chairs.

Reducing length of utterance, linguistic complexity and improving semantic contingency

Parents may use language which is too sophisticated for the child's level of functioning or is not relevant to the child's conversation or activity.

Relevance to child's fluency

Research has shown that if a child attempts longer or more complex utterances his fluency is more likely to break down. If the parents are using sophisticated language, the child may try to match the parents' level and experience fluency failure. Using language that is not semantically contingent interrupts the child's processing of language and introduces cognitive and linguistic material unrelated to his thoughts or activities, this puts the child's language and fluency under pressure.

Techniques to achieve change

The parents are guided towards using short utterances with simple vocabulary. It is helpful to use language that refers to the 'here and now', for example:

Child:	the daddy sleeps in this bed.
Parent:	yes, he's tired Goodnight daddy

as opposed to:

Child:	the daddy sleeps in this bed.
Parent:	I'm putting this chair in the sitting room. It's just like the one in grandma's house — you know the one with the orange cushion on it.

Reducing questions

Parents may attempt to engage a child and encourage conversation by asking a series of questions (some of which may not even require an answer) without allowing the child adequate time to respond.

Relevance to child's fluency

Research has indicated that a child's fluency is under greatest pressure when responding to questions, especially open questions.

Techniques to achieve change

Parents are encouraged to find alternatives to questions. Making comments on the child's and their own activity can be helpful and research has shown that commenting facilitates communication with children more effectively than the use of questions. However, some parents find this difficult initially and may need time to discuss and practise this skill.

Improving language input

Occasionally a parent's conversation with the child lacks content, is vague and overuses deixis, for example, *'Put that thing here and I'll put the other one on top, this can go there — by that one.'*

Relevance to child's fluency

The fluency of some children appears to be affected by an impoverished vocabulary or a specific word retrieval difficulty. Helping parents develop skills that have been shown to enrich the child's lexicon and language skills, may also assist in the stabilisation of the child's fluency.

Techniques to achieve change

Parents are encouraged to use the right labels for the play material, adding descriptive words, such as adjectives and adverbs, as appropriate. For example, *'I'll put my blue car in the petrol station' 'I've parked it behind the taxi'*.

The parent's level of complexity may need monitoring in order to avoid putting the child's fluency at risk.

Improving reinforcement

Some parents have difficulty responding positively to the child's utterances or actions. The verbal reinforcers may include 'mm' 'yeah' 'uh hah' 'really' and the non-verbal behaviours, such as smiling, facial expressions, nodding the head.

Relevance to child's fluency

Research has shown that fluency is adversely affected by a negative parental style.

Techniques to achieve change

The clinician may find a brainstorm with the parents will help provide several ways of responding positively. Parents are encouraged to respond to all the child's comments or questions, and if they do not know what to say in response, they may find it helpful to repeat what the child has said in a confirmatory style for example:

Child: 'my man's riding on this horse.'
Parents: 'yes, your man's riding on that horse.'

Further positive commenting on the child's actions should be encouraged, for example, *'I see you have put all those pigs in the field, now they are safe, that was a good idea'*. Parents should be encouraged to be specific and descriptive in their positive statements, as in the example, rather than resorting to generalised praise, e.g. *'Good boy'*, *'You are clever'*. A more detailed discussion of praise and reinforcement will be found in Chapter 7. A case study is included here as an illustration of some of the issues raised in this chapter.

Case Study

Carly, aged 3;2, attended for assessment and treatment of her dysfluency which was characterised by prolongations and struggle behaviour. Her speech and language skills were within normal limits.

During the interview her parents, James and Kim, described her early years as traumatic, beginning with her premature birth at 29 weeks followed by incubation and ventilation for several weeks. Carly had several convulsions, suffered recurrent urinary tract infections and was regularly unwell with minor illnesses. Her parents had received instructions on how to revive Carly should she stop breathing during convulsion. There was, therefore, considerable anxiety about her wellbeing and Carly had never been left in the care of anybody else. At the time of the interview Carly was still sleeping in the parents' bed at night, and had not yet begun attending nursery school.

Assessment of parent–child interaction revealed that James tended to ask frequent questions without waiting for a response. He also spoke very rapidly and quietly. Kim used a moderate rate of speech but hardly paused between utterances, giving Carly very little time to respond or initiate.

A 6-week course of therapy was arranged. The Special Time task was set, although both parents commented that they did little else but play with Carly on her own. However, after the first week they reported that the Special Times had a different quality to their usual time with her. Interaction therapy commenced: James quickly identified his habit of asking questions, Kim, on the other hand, needed some guidance in order to identify her tendency to talk without pausing. James spent three weeks working on reducing questions as he found this very difficult, especially if Carly was not talkative. However, he began to develop other strategies, using humour and commenting to engage Carly. Once he had consolidated this style his rapid rate of speech was targeted and he was able to reduce this with relative ease. Kim worked hard at increasing pausing and although she reported that it felt very unnatural, once having mastered this skill she felt it was important to adopt this style not only during Special Times but also at times throughout the day with Carly. A byproduct of the increased pausing was that her general rate of speech was reduced and the pace of her interactional style became more compatible with that of Carly.

At the fourth therapy appointment the subject of Carly's sleeping habit was raised with the intention of suggesting some changes. However, James and Kim reported that following the formulation of the assessment when it was suggested that the high levels of interdependence at night might become problematic, they had discussed the matter and decided to involve Carly in the planning and decorating of a bedroom for her so that she could move in. They had completed the decoration and were just about to start the moving process. During the next two therapy sessions this was reviewed and discussed.

Carly's dysfluency was variable during the 6 weeks of therapy but a pattern emerged. Carly was very fluent during the week, with a deterioration marked by prolongations during Sunday. This was discussed and seemed to be linked to Carly's anxiety about attending nursery on a Monday, which she had started at the same time as therapy commenced. James and Kim were given literature to read on *How to help your child express his feelings* (Faber and Mazlish, 1980). They then explored how they might recognise Carly's emotions and help her to express them.

After the 6 weeks of therapy, James and Kim maintained the Special Time task throughout the consolidation period, as well as implementing other suggestions. Carly's fluency improved during this period with two exceptions. On one occasion the family had a busy weekend with late nights. By the Monday Carly's dysfluency had markedly deteriorated. Her parents reinstated the earlier bedtimes and the usual routine, including the Special Times, and Carly's fluency stabilised. Two weeks later Carly became ill and, once again, her dysfluency increased. Kim and James kept up the Special Times and ensured Carly was getting extra sleep with no other demands on her. As soon as her health was restored, so Carly's fluency was re-established.

Carly's progress continued to be monitored. She has occasional lapses in fluency, usually associated with illness but her parents confidently manage these such that she is quickly stabilised again. The periods of dysfluency tend to be shorter in duration and with increasingly longer intervals inbetween. The family will be monitored until all parties are satisfied that no further input is required. James and Kim are now able to express their confidence in dealing with Carly's fluency and its ups and downs.

Summary

The format of this approach is consistent with the research findings identified in the previous chapter. We have described the process of interaction therapy, including the use of video recordings to help parents identify, change and monitor their patterns of interaction in order to facilitate the child's fluency. This therapeutic approach provides parents with the skills and resources necessary to overcome the feelings of helplessness that are so often apparent at the beginning of therapy. Thus empowered, the parents are more able to manage further episodes of dysfluency with equanimity.

Chapter 7
Family Issues

Introduction

We have described an interactionist model for stuttering which provides a framework within which each child and family present with a different configuration of variables that are likely to affect the dysfluency problem. These are identified during the assessment and interview procedures for each family. There is to date no proven formula for deciding which of these variables are the key issues for a particular child or family so the clinician must rely on knowledge and experience to set up hypotheses and test them out in therapy. There is considerable research and literature available to support therapy targeted at parent–child interaction styles and direct speech modification. However, there may be other issues that the therapist identified during the Formulation procedure as being of concern to the family. Commonly these include childhood tantrums, bedtime routines, sibling rivalry, and inconsistent management.

There is a general consensus in the literature that these issues are related to the dysfluency and would be included amongst the emotional/environmental factors described earlier. Glasner (1970) emphasised the child's interpersonal relationships in the family as primary in the development of the problem. Moore and Nystul (1979) examined parent–child attitudes and the communication processes within families with a stuttering member, and found evidence of specific maladjustment, concluding that parent attitudes are paramount in constituting the nature of the home environment. Bloodstein (1987; 1995) also reported that a sizeable proportion of the parents of stutterers appear to be in varying degrees 'demanding' 'over anxious' or 'perfectionist' in their child-rearing practices. Riley and Riley (1983) found half their sample of parents had high expectations of their children.

Prins (1983) indicated several sources of environmental stresses including erratic planning and conduct of daily routines, time pressures, unpredictable changes in the household, behavioural demands the child cannot meet and insufficient individual time with the child. It is clear, therefore, that these issues cannot be ignored and that any comprehensive package of therapy should address them. We would, however, share the view expressed by Hayhow and Levy (1989) that 'we should not attempt to make all families orderly, predictable and child centred' but rather, having identified those issues of concern to the family, help them explore and experiment with alternative strategies and, ultimately, assist them in making productive changes. It is our intention throughout therapy to help parents regain confidence in their skills and abilities, enabling them to find their own solutions to the difficulties that arise. Clinicians may find that as interaction therapy progresses, parents take the initiative and begin to problem-solve on their own, using the clinician perhaps as a 'sounding board' or reinforcer. For some families the number of issues identified at the assessment may diminish rapidly whilst for others it may take longer but the process remains the same.

The issues presented by families are infinite in their variability. However, there are some which in our experience appear to be common to many, we have divided these into two groups: environmental and emotional, and it is these we shall discuss in this chapter.

Environmental issues

Reactions to dysfluency

Wendell Johnson's (Johnson, 1959) Diagnosogenic Theory put forward the view that parents' verbal and non-verbal reactions to a child's dysfluency may be responsible for stuttering. Since that time much of the commonly accepted advice given to parents has been that they should not draw attention to it and it would go away. Although this advice has been helpful to some parents and children, there are those for whom it was not. To assume that the same advice will be appropriate for all dysfluent children ignores the evidence which clearly demonstrates the heterogeneity of the disorder. It also denies the natural instinct of many parents to assist a child who is having difficulties. Parents have described the distress and anxiety they have experienced whilst trying to ignore the lengthy strugglings of their once fluent child. One mother reported, *'I try so hard to look as if nothing has happened but inside I feel so awful and I'm sure it must show'*. Some parents find their wish to talk about the dysfluency is so great that they invent a secret code to enable them to do so. We quoted an example in Chapter 4 where the parents referred to the child's dysfluency as 'the car'. This allowed the parents to deal with their anxiety but left the child utterly confused as he was aware that the family did not own a car.

Most parents faced with a child experiencing difficulties will instinctively go to his assistance. For example, they might pick up a child that has fallen over, offering help and advice as they do so; the child expects the parents to behave in this manner, but finds that when he is having similar difficulties with his talking, it is ignored and never mentioned. In our experience most households have few subjects that are unmentionable. Issues such as sex, money, or divorce are, with the exception of some cultural and religious groups, discussed as appropriate. If a child's dysfluency becomes the only subject that cannot be discussed then it assumes a gravity and importance beyond all proportion. There are, indeed, many adults in therapy who have never mentioned their stutter to anyone apart from perhaps a speech therapist. The strength of this conspiracy of silence is compelling and has been maintained by many professionals and by society generally.

It is not our intention to create a problem where one does not exist. However, we do consider that it is our role to encourage parents to maintain an open dialogue with their child about their speech, just as they would with any other problem, especially where a child is showing an awareness of the dysfluency. Many parents we have interviewed have acted upon the advice they have received and ignored the child's speech difficulties and as a result believe the child is unaware of the dysfluency. As part of the assessment, children are routinely asked to comment on their speech (see Chapter 3) many of whom are able to describe the problem clearly and eloquently often to the surprise of their parents. There are also children who are observed changing words which are difficult, stamping their feet or putting their hands over their mouths, all of which are strategies the children employ in an attempt to speak more fluently. It is arguable that all these children are also demonstrating a level of awareness of their dysfluency. In our clinical experience many of these children and their parents benefited from being able to talk about their speech. Acknowledging difficulties and talking about them seems to lessen the associated feelings of anxiety. It is clearly very important, however, that the advice given by therapists is tailored to the individual needs of each child and their family.

Parents frequently seek advice on the management of the child's dysfluency early in the assessment process and therapists should resist the temptation to give advice before the procedures are complete. On completion of all the assessments the therapist will be in a position to make an informed decision as to the most appropriate advice. As a rule, however, parents should be encouraged to acknowledge the difficulty of a child who is clearly aware of the dysfluency. They may find it helpful to experiment with comments, such as *'Oh dear, that was a bit hard for you to say wasn't it?'* *'You know I think you had so much to say it just got stuck on the way'*. Or, *'I think we're both in too much of a hurry I'm going to go slowly lets see if that helps'*. These comments allow parents to be sympathetic, offer explanations or advice in the same way they may have done for many other problems. We have known parents for whom permission to acknowledge the difficulty has in itself resulted in such a decrease in anxiety that a reduction in dysfluency was noted before interaction therapy began. Developing an open dialogue between therapists, parents and children is fundamental to our approach. Parents are seen as the experts in their children and therapy as a process in which therapists facilitate parents in making small self-determined changes in their interactive style. Enabling parents to experiment with alternative ways of managing the dysfluency is often the first step in this process.

Routines

We have mentioned previously that structuring a consistent and predictable routine appears to be helpful to children who are dysfluent while disruptions in the normal and expected pattern of events will often result in increased dysfluency. Transitions from school to holiday time may cause problems, and parents who are aware of these potential difficulties can assist by finding ways of helping the child adjust from one situation to another.

During the interview parents often describe the deleterious effect of excitement on the child's fluency. The gradual build up towards Christmas is often a particularly difficult time for parents to contain the level of excitement. Schools, relatives, the media, parties and visits from Father Christmas all have a contribution to make to the rising levels of anticipation. Parents therefore have an important role in maintaining the normal routines of home and exerting a calming influence on their children.

Birthdays and family holidays offer similar opportunity for a gradual build up of anticipatory delight and parents need to discuss how they might manage these in the future in such a way as to minimise negative effects. Families have found it helpful to ensure that routines such as children's bedtimes are not unduly disturbed, and that the dysfluent child in particular is not allowed to become overtired, as parents report that this will often disrupt fluency. If Special Times have been established (see Chapter 6) it is particularly important that they are maintained at these times. Parents often find this difficult but can be reminded that for most children this is an essential part of fluency stabilisation. A parent may contact the clinic, distressed that the child's fluency has deteriorated and after some discussion it becomes apparent that the Special Times have lapsed. This often occurs because of the general disruption to routine, but is sometimes curtailed as a result of the child becoming fluent. Reinstatement of the Special Times may, in some cases, be sufficient to restore fluency.

Turn-taking

Various responses to questions during the parent interview will indicate if there is some difficulty in taking turns to talk within the family. There may be several children competing with one another to have their say, or the household may comprise mostly adults, for example, parents, plus grandparents, au pairs, etc. with the child being far outnumbered. Either scenario may result in the dysfluent child having insufficient opportunity to speak without fear of interruption by another person. Alternatively, the dysfluent child may be monopolising family conversations, talking in lengthy monologues with everyone else being reluctant to interrupt in case the dysfluency increases. In either case, it is essential to redress the balance so that each family member is allowed sufficient time and space to have their say without being interrupted or pressurised to hurry and finish speaking.

In order to improve turn-taking skills, it is first necessary for the parents to understand the present system operating within their family. We frequently use an observation exercise which both parents undertake and report back separately.

Exercise

When your family is all together, for example at a meal time, observe them and write down the following:

- Who does the most talking?
- Who does the most listening?
- Who does the most interrupting?

The parents do not need to reach a consensus on their observations, rather to consider their own role and the role of other family members in the turn-taking system. They record their observations which are then discussed during the next treatment session.

After the parents have reported their findings, a discussion regarding the value of turn-taking and its role in the management of the dysfluent child should include the following points.

Balanced turn-taking ensures that:

- The dysfluent child knows he will have a turn to talk without the extra pressure of having to break in.
- The dysfluent child is able to finish what he is saying without fear of being interrupted before he has finished.
- Other family members have the opportunity to speak.
- No one can interrupt or be interrupted unless someone is rambling on too long.
- There are no 'pay offs' in being dysfluent.

When parents have understood the importance of turn-taking it may be helpful to suggest the following exercise in order to establish a more appropriate pattern.

Exercise

Find a microphone — it may be a real one or a toy — and when the family is together instruct everybody that only the person holding the microphone is allowed to speak. Lay the microphone in the middle of the table, instruct everyone that when they wish to speak they should pick it up and speak. When they have finished they pass it to the next person who has a contribution to make or replace it on the table. Nobody is allowed to speak unless they have the microphone.

It may be helpful to begin with a story that everyone contributes to: *'One day as I was walking down the'* ... (next person) *'railway line I met an old man'* ... next, etc. This establishes the idea of turn-taking, following which the family can have a conversation passing the microphone around, with one of the parents ensuring that each member has a fair chance to speak.

This exercise may only need to be undertaken a few times, provided that everyone has understood the principle. In our experience, children as young as 2 years are able to participate fully. Once the idea of turn-taking has been understood the use of the microphone rapidly becomes unnecessary, but it can be referred to, for example, *'John don't interrupt, Michael has the microphone'*.

Choice of nursery/school

Parents may seek advice concerning a suitable nursery or school placement for the dysfluent child. In our experience, certain aspects of a nursery or school environment would seem to enhance fluency so we generally make the following recommendations:

- The child may feel more settled and calm in an environment where there is a routine which enables the child to predict what will happen and therefore feel more in control.
- The child would benefit from a classroom situation where there is less competition for the adult's attention, a higher adult:child ratio and a system of turn-taking to speak.
- A school which places great emphasis on academic achievement may be a difficult and pressured environment for the child, thus putting the fluency at greater risk.
- The parents may wish to find out about the school's management of problems, such as children teasing one another, as this might be a potential issue for their child.

A discussion of this nature is often instigated by parents and usually occurs where parents are concerned about the suitability of the child's current placement, or where a move is under consideration. The points described above may be useful to consider during the session.

Working with parents who have a first language other than English

A survey of speech and language therapists in Britain working with British Asian children who stutter reveals that many judge their work with this client group to be less successful (Wright and Sherrard, 1994). This highlights the need to explore alternative or modified therapeutic models in response to specific needs. As argued by one Health Authority, 'Providing the same service to all in the face of differing needs is not an equitable service' (Wandsworth and East Merton Health Authority, 1979).

Providing an effective service transculturally raises a number of issues and challenges which require a creative and flexible approach from the clinician:

- There is a need to establish a sound understanding of the clients' culture and how this might influence their perception of the syndrome of stuttering, along with the expectations of therapy.
- In addition, studies indicate that cultural differences exist in terms of parenting styles, caregiver–child discourse and communicative expectations (Taylor and Clarke, 1994).
- It is generally accepted that there are inherent difficulties in establishing and maintaining effective communication when therapist and client do not share a common language. We have observed that inadequate communication is more likely to occur with parents who have a first language other than English, despite the use of trained interpreters.
- It is also apparent that these parents often have less opportunity to seek clarification during therapy or may be reluctant to do so. Nadirshaw (1993) points out that good communication plays a key role in maintaining the therapeutic relationship, and predicts where this is not achieved, there is a subsequent negative effect on therapy outcomes. Nelson-Jones (1988) suggests that having clear goals positively influences the degree to which clients persevere with therapeutic tasks.
- It has also been found that clients from ethnic communities may experience difficulty in attending a centre that is not within or nearby their community. Fear of racial abuse or attack may inhibit travelling within areas known to be overly racist or hostile. A local survey highlights the less frequent use of health services by Bengali and Chinese men and suggests that this could also influence the clients' ability to commit themselves to the standard requirement of both parents attending.
- It is also important for therapists to be aware that clients may approach therapy with previously negative experience of health services that are insensitive to cultural differences and racial issues.

Subsequent low expectations on the part of the client may be reenforced when a service appears foreign or intimidating. D'Ardenne and Mahtani (1989) discuss how use of the clients' own language signals respect.

It is in response to these factors that we are in the process of developing and adapting our interaction programme for use in translation. The package will be presented in the parents' first language, thus facilitating accurate communication of general information as well as specific instructions between the clinician and the family.

As a precurser to translation, community members have been consulted to help us ensure that the material provided is culturally appropriate and relevant. To date the programme has been distributed to members of the Urdu-speaking Moslem community for review, their comments have been received and changes made as appropriate in response.

Our initial conclusions are that for parents who are highly motivated, and accustomed to obtaining information from the written word, use of this programme in a self-help capacity can effect positive change. Decrease in parental anxiety related to having information about stuttering, better understanding of the problem, and positive strategies to implement is noted, along with the ability of some parents to achieve change in their interactional style independently. However, it is apparent that self-help is not an approach that is universally helpful, and it is felt that for many parents, a written programme such as this, would be best used in conjunction with therapist support. Concerns are also felt about the degree to which parents from ethnic communities are able to access the written word. Davis and Aslam (1981) refer to a survey in Birmingham following the translation of material into three Asian languages. It found that 80% of those taking part in the survey were not literate in their first language and, furthermore, those that were literate in their first language were also literate in English. Tape recording the programme will enable families with literacy difficulties to access the information independently.

This approach affords greater flexibility, the opportunity to enhance therapist–client communication, and could make a useful contribution to the provision of a culturally sensitive service. Use of the parents' language should also help convey the clinician's acceptance and validation of the parents' cultural background. Furthermore, the written format will provide a clear outline of therapy goals, thus encouraging the parents' motivation in treatment.

The package will be suitable for use in the clinical setting or as a home programme under the clinician's supervision. Either approach offers more flexibility, as clinic attendance may involve one parent who takes the material home to their partner, or another member of the family or community may participate. D'Ardenne and Mahtani (1989) stress the importance of family and community networks and encourage counsellors to consider ways of involving them. If attendance is problematic the programme could be carried out in the stuttering child's home with the clinician corresponding via an interpreter with the parents.

In order to address the issue of the clinician's understanding of the parents' culture, their perception of the stuttering problem, and their expectations of therapy, it is essential that the comprehensive assessment of the child and family is undertaken. The parent interview will necessarily involve the use of trained interpreters which will inevitably make it a more lengthy process. However, it is perhaps even more crucial that clinicians have a thorough understanding of the child and the family systems in a culture which is unfamiliar to them.

The programme currently being piloted is presented with an introduction followed by a schedule of tasks for parents to complete. The introduction contains four sections dealing, respectively, with the nature of stuttering, generally agreed facts about stuttering, how to respond to stuttering behaviour, and how to talk about stuttering. We have found the latter to be a difficult area for many parents, particularly when they have been advised by relatives or other health professionals to 'ignore' their child's stutter. Examples are given of appropriate responses which aim to help break the frequently held 'conspiracy of silence' which ensues. In our experience the relief for both parents and child when the problem is acknowledged can have a positive effect on fluency. As described by one parent:

> *'I cannot explain the relief this has given to our son. He seems to have visibly relaxed, appears so much more content, and his speech over the last week has improved dramatically.'*

The second section of the programme consists of an eight-step schedule for parents to implement over 2 months. Each step discusses one aspect of interaction and instructs parents how to modify their interactional style.

Goals have been selected in accordance with the features of parental interaction which we have identified as being significant, and which we have found to feature most frequently in our assessments.

Bilingualism

Some of the children we have seen in clinic are exposed to more than one language within the home environment. This extra demand placed on a vulnerable child's developing system may be contributing to the dysfluency. Temporarily reducing the number of linguistic systems to which the child is responding may prove helpful. It is important for the family to understand the rationale for this action, as the choice of language will be important, and should be that most commonly used by all members of the household. Where this arrangement is not possible it is important to consider consistency of language use, so that the child can identify and predict the language he might hear from the various people with whom he communicates. One family we saw spoke Yiddish at home, English at school and also used Hebrew from time to time.

Case Example

> Esther, who was 4 years old, had been delayed in her acquisition of language, and had recently become dysfluent. She had just started school and was being exposed to English for the first time. After discussing the issues with her parents (both of whom are fluent in (Yiddish and English) it was decided that they would establish Yiddish at home consistently. Up until that time both parents and other children in the household used a mixture of Yiddish and English, often switching mid-sentence. This was one of a number of changes made during therapy but was instrumental in providing a stable and consistent language environment at home and resulted in improvements in Esther's expressive language skills particularly as regards her vocabulary. Once Esther's fluency had been stable for some months the family adopted a more flexible approach to the use of language at home with no ill effect. Esther, however, continued to use Yiddish consistently at home and English in school.

Emotional issues

Managing behaviour

In our experience, the families of stuttering children are very rarely disturbed or dysfunctional. Their child-rearing practices may be no different to their own experience of being parented and may be similar to many other families. However, the environment they have created may not be helpful to a child who is vulnerable to fluency breakdown. It is important that parents understand this point of view in order to minimise guilt and prevent them beginning to, or continuing to construe themselves as inadequate. Discussions of these more general issues should be carefully timed and is often best after some of the interaction therapy sessions have taken place. The parents will have begun to discover that small changes in their behaviour will have a direct effect on the child and his speech. In addition, the parents will have achieved these changes by viewing themselves objectively, a process that can also be used to help them re–evaluate more general management issues.

Consistency has often been highlighted as an issue for parents, and may be responsible for many problems within the family. Parents often mean to be consistent but may find themselves backing down or changing the ground rules which causes confusion within the family. The first step may simply be to facilitate a discussion between the parents as to why being inconsistent is counterproductive. Helping parents to establish a few simple rules within the household and supporting each other in upholding them may be necessary before any other issues can be discussed. It will also be important for the parents to discuss their anxieties about the effect that these steps may have on the child's dysfluency. We have seen many parents where the child's level of dysfluency is the criteria for management, rather than the child's behaviour, and this can result in a situation in which the dysfluency begins to have 'pay offs' (Perkins 1992). Parents become so fearful of upsetting the dysfluent child that they may apply a different set of rules to him.

Case Example

> This was particularly true of one family with a strong family history of stuttering, whose eldest son, aged 9, was already in treatment and whose youngest daughter, then aged 3, became very dysfluent over a period of 2 months. She was prolonging vowels and showing signs of struggle behaviour, putting her hand over her mouth and stamping her foot. The parents became very distressed and anxious. Further discussions established that they were having difficulties managing her behaviour which had deteriorated along with the dysfluency. They had begun to treat her differently from the other children in order to try and reduce the dysfluency. As the boundaries they set on her behaviour became increasingly blurred, so the anxiety levels increased, and with it the dysfluency. Helping the parents to reinstate the boundaries of acecptable behaviour restored the equilibrium of the family, consequently, the child's behaviour became more manageable, and the dysfluency reduced.

When parents begin to look at these issues, it is often helpful for them to set aside a time in the week where they will talk about the management of the children, during this time difficult situations that have arisen can be discussed and decisions taken about how to manage similar events in future. It is also a time when parents can reinforce and support each other in their attempts to change what they are doing.

Praise and reinforcement

Branden (1972) states that in his view there is no value judgement more important to man, no factor more decisive in his psychological development and motivation than the estimate he attributes to himself. He continues, stating that the nature of a person's self-evaluation has profound effects on his thinking process, emotions, desires, values and goals, and it is the single most significant key to his behaviour.

Helping parents to find successful ways of praising and reinforcing their dysfluent children has always been an integral part of our therapeutic approach (Rustin, 1987; Rustin and Kuhr, 1989). Parents whose self-esteem is low and whose own parenting did not include reinforcement may find it particularly difficult to praise their own children. It is important to provide clear guidelines for parents whose lack of experience will make it difficult for them to succeed on their own. Many parents report that they do praise their children, but closer observation and monitoring may reveal that it is infrequent, non-contingent, insincere, sarcastic or followed by a statement that negates it, for example, *'Clever boy you tidied up your toys — why don't you always do it like that?'*.

Clinicians may find it helpful to ask parents to monitor how and when they praise the child and write it down for discussion during the following treatment session. Dr Haim Ginott (1969) suggests that helpful praise comes in three parts:

- The adult describes with appreciation what they see or feel, for example, *'Well done Philip, you came straightaway when I called you for breakfast'*.
- They should then offer the child an adjective to describe the action or the activity, e.g. *'That was very helpful/thoughtful/kind of you'*.
- The child, after hearing the description and finding it to be true, is then able to accept it and, ultimately, apply the description to himself, for example, *'Yes, I am helpful'*.

Case Example

A child presented her mother with a painting, which was a series of colourful scribbles. Instead of saying, *'Oh, that's beautiful'* (a remark that was not really accurate) the mother said, *'I really like the pink swirl and that bit that goes round and round you must have worked very hard at it'*, the child responded by saying *'Yes I did and I'm going to do another one'* and thus encouraged by her efforts she went on to do just that.

The effect of this approach to praise giving is that children receive reinforcement from an adult and are then able to apply it to themselves. Once this skill is learnt in childhood it will stand them in good stead for the rest of their lives. The above parent explained that previously when faced with the child's paintings she had responded with *'Oh that's beautiful/well done'* only to have the child reply *'No its not, its rubbish. I can't paint'* and throw it in the bin. It is important to give parents examples of how to praise and to assist them in making a list of the things their child does that warrants praise. Further practical examples can be found in *How to Talk so Kids will Listen and Listen so Kids Will Talk* (Faber and Mazlish, 1980).

Finally, parents may find it helpful to be given specific homework targets which the clinician can then monitor and shape. For example, each parent identifies one thing to praise every day and records:

- What the child did or said that the parent wishes to praise.
- What the parent said when praising the child.
- How the child responded.

This should continue until the parents are satisfied that they are able to praise regularly and successfully. Once the effects on the child's behaviour become noticeable, the parents are, in turn, reinforced by the evidence of their own success. It is helpful to include the whole family in this process, with the parents, acting as role models, to demonstrate how to give praise to others as well as how to receive it positively.

Sleeping

Parents report that the three most difficult problems to cope with are sleeping, eating and speech. The infant needs to sleep, and when it cries it is commonly the mother's role to comfort the child and take care of its needs so that it will sleep. A fretful child who does not sleep could reinforce a mother's feelings of inadequacy, exacerbating her own tiredness and anxiety and leaving her less able to cope with a crying baby. It is therefore no surprise that manageable routines for bedtimes and sleeping are difficult to establish, and that the problems described by parents are very variable. These include children who are unsettled, wake up frequently, sleep in the parental bed, or refuse to go to bed without their siblings. Although it is not possible to set hard and fast rules about how to manage these situations, the therapist can help parents become more creative in finding solutions that are likely to have a successful outcome. This will, of course, depend on the age of the child, the nature of the difficulty and the parents' management style. We have found a problem-solving approach is often very helpful as it allows the parents to be very active in seeking their own solutions (Rustin, 1987; Rustin and Kuhr, 1989). Briefly, this requires the parents to describe the problem in some detail, to isolate the problem and write it in the middle of a sheet of paper. Parents and therapist then 'brainstorm' as many potential solutions as they can think of, without making any judgements as to their suitability. When all ideas are exhausted then those already attempted and found unhelpful are ruled out, leaving several new ideas that might provide a solution. These are then explored in terms of the predicted outcomes and ranked in order, the first being that which is considered most likely to succeed. The first solution should then be discussed fully, its execution planned and then attempted as part of the homework for the following week. Solutions that parents have found helpful include:

- Negotiating separate bedtimes according to age.
- Abandoning a daytime sleep.
- Star charts with a reward system.

- Setting a bedtime routine.
- Asking the child to describe what he needs in order to comply, for example, a nightlight or a clock.

Case Example

Moses was 2½, had suffered from colic and had always been difficult to settle. At the time of assessment there was no set time or routine for bedtime. He would fall asleep on the sofa eventually between 10–11 pm. This left no time for the parents and was placing considerable strain on their relationship.

Moses went to a childminder most days who was allowing him to sleep at midday for 2–3 hours. A variety of alternatives was discussed, and the final solution involved talking to the childminder and making arrangements for her to eliminate the midday sleep. Concurrently, the family established a routine that involved bathtime, storytime, drink and bed at a predetermined time, 6.30 in this case. The childminder was very cooperative and kept Moses awake and entertained. He was so tired by 6.30 pm he fell asleep during the story. Praise and reinforcement ensured this pattern was maintained.

In some cases it will be necessary for the parents to discuss the problem with the whole family, sharing with them the new arrangements that will be put in place. It is important that each family member understands the role they have to play in facilitating the changes so that they can share in the success.

Case Example

Harry, aged 4, who was dysfluent, had a brother Rory, aged 6, and a sister Amy, aged 2. This was a busy and unstructured household and it was difficult to get the children into bed before 9.30 pm. The parents decided that Harry's bedtime should be at 7.00 and that Rory should be allowed to stay up until 7.30 while Amy should be in bed by 6.30. This established a hierarchy for the children's bedtime and ensured that Harry had sufficient sleep. It also required the parents to discuss at some length the routines required to implement these changes. They had some difficulty establishing this bedtime regime, but it was finally achieved after several weeks, much to the parents' satisfaction.

Eating

One of the first and most important functions a mother has is to feed her infant. Anything that interferes with her ability to perform this function undermines her sense of worth as a mother. Bloodstein (1987) suggests that regular sleeping and eating habits can influence a child's dysfluency. However, eating — like sleeping — can become a battleground for parents. The children may have to be coerced into eating, refuse to eat, eat very little, demand snacks, take excessively long to eat or just become very fussy and will only eat certain things, such as ice cream and bread.

Once again the solutions will depend to some extent upon the family and the circumstances. However, the therapist will be able to employ similar problem-solving strategies to those suggested for sleeping problems.

Case Example

Adam was 4 years old, stubborn and disinterested in food. He would eventually eat but it would take a very long time. His mother would alternately scold, threaten, bribe and coerce him. A brainstorm of the problem produced several solutions that could be combined:

- Give smaller amounts on the plate to increase the chances of success and rewards for eating his food.
- A time limit set on how long was reasonable for him to sit with the food in front of him, after which the food would be removed.
- Warn the child that it would be taken away in 5 minutes.
- The food would be removed at the appointed time and thrown away.
- There would be no snack foods between meals.
- Tell the child what they were going to do at each stage.
- The parents would set aside 10 minutes at the end of the day to discuss how they were managing.

They felt it was important to encourage each other when it went well, and to work out what had gone wrong if it had not been successful. The parents went away not convinced they could manage it. However, they decided to begin at the weekend in order that they could support each other. Adam's mother found it very difficult to allow him to eat less initially, but soon discovered that if he did not eat much at one meal, and there were no snacks in between, then the child often ate all the food (smaller portions) and more at the next. It took 2 weeks to establish this new regime and they were delighted with their success.

Sleeping and eating problems seem to occur quite frequently amongst the families we have seen. There are, however, other issues which appear less often but are nonetheless important.

Illness

In our experience, a child's fluency level is directly affected by his physical wellbeing, and any illness causes a temporary relapse in progress. Parents should be made aware of the inevitability of this occurring and advised on how best to manage it. Parents should ensure that the child is getting sufficient sleep to overcome the illness. If Special Times have been abandoned, they should be resumed as soon as the child is well enough. Normal routines should be reinstated as soon as possible.

However, illness may occur in a sibling, parent or other close relative. Parents instinctively wish to protect their children from difficult, painful or unpleasant situations, however, this is often either not possible, not practical, or unhelpful. It has always been our policy to encourage parents to share the concerns of the family with the child at a level appropriate for their age. If therefore someone is ill, they should provide simple explanations of what the problem is and what is likely to happen. They should also attempt to verbalise some of the feelings that the child may be experiencing, allowing them to feel afraid or upset. Children like adults respond best when they are listened to, accepted and understood. Similarly, talking things through is the most helpful way of relieving anxiety and at their own level children are no exception to this rule.

Parents often imagine they can protect children from the pain and sadness of illness but are usually mistaken, as children are often painfully aware that something is wrong but without any more information often blame themselves for the parents' distress.

Case Example

One parent contacted the clinic as the child, who had been fluent for some time, had recently become dysfluent. After some discussion it was revealed that the grandmother had been taken ill and was in hospital. The family were very concerned about her, but had chosen to keep the news from the child as he was very attached to her, and they were anxious not to upset him as it might disrupt his fluency. The parents came to the clinic to discuss the issues raised and as a result decided to tell the child what had happened and explain how anxious and worried they had been. Later the child drew a picture for his grandmother and asked if he could visit her, this was discussed at some length and a visit arranged for the following week. The parents kept in touch by phone and were finally able to report that the fluency had returned to its previous level.

Changes and loss

Major changes in the household present similar problems. Moving house; change in caregivers (childminders, nannies, etc.); changes in marital relationship; divorce; separation; death; all involve degrees of loss.

Bereavement

For many parents their ability to deal successfully with bereavement and loss is often dependant on their own experience of death. Therapists can refer to the parental interview for evidence of bereavement and the strategies used for dealing with it. Some parents feel strongly that death is something children should be protected from and may develop elaborate stories to explain the sudden death of a family member.

Case Example

A child whose much loved grandfather died suddenly was told he had 'gone away'. The child was left feeling upset and confused as to why his grandfather should have suddenly gone away and wondered if he had done something wrong. He was also unable to make sense of his mother's emotional swings while mourning the loss of her father.

As in previous examples our advice to parents has been to talk to children at a level they can understand. They should share with them the circumstances surrounding the loss and what will happen as a result. Children need to understand the feelings they may experience and parents should share their own sadness with their child. Teaching children how to deal with death can often begin with the death of a much loved pet. For many children this is a difficult experience. However, it provides an opportunity to help the child understand the meaning of death. Parents should encourage the child to be upset, to cry and talk about the feelings they have. The child may wish to talk about the loved pet for some time before a replacement can be considered, and the pace is best decided by the child. A similar approach can be employed when dealing with a death in the family. Talking about the event and the circumstances, sharing feelings, and allowing time for the process of bereavement to run its course is very important for all concerned, we would recommend ***Death in the Family*** (Pincus, 1976) and ***Grief in Children*** (Dryregrov, 1990) for further reading.

Moving house

Stress scales such as that of Holmes and Rahe (1967) place moving house high on the list of stressors within families. However, parents often underestimate the emotional and physical impact it has on their children. One child became very distressed as he thought he was being left behind with the house. He had understood that it was ***his parents*** who were moving as they had said *'We're moving'*. This highlights the necessity of keeping the child informed of what is occurring, and in helping him prepare for the event. There are, in addition, practical steps that can be taken, such as allowing the child to choose the familiar items he wants to take from the old house to the new one, allowing the children to negotiate which rooms will be theirs, perhaps even the colour it should be painted, etc. It may also be possible to involve them in some of the choices associated with making the new purchase, to allow them to see around the new area, find out about the amenities that are available, and compare these with the old one.

Change of caregiver

Where new caregivers, such as nannies or childminders, are to be appointed, keeping the child informed is essential and, if appropriate, his opinion may also be sought. But perhaps most importantly the child needs to feel that the loved nanny, childminder, or au pair who is leaving will not abandon him. It would be helpful for the child and caregiver to keep in touch, to visit, telephone or write and perhaps leave a photograph. This will help the child appreciate that he is still loved by the absent adult despite the physical separation.

Divorce/separation

As many as one in three families will experience divorce or separation. It is therefore a situation that therapists will be presented with frequently. If during the interview, it has become apparent that the parents are experiencing difficulties in their relationship, therapists may find it necessary to refer the family for appropriate counselling.

Increasingly, parents are either divorced, living apart or in the process of separation. The issue for clinicians will then be how best to help the parents organise themselves in such a way as to minimise the effects on the child. Clinicians are in a position to provide the opportunity for the parents to discuss with each other, in the presence of a third party, how they might be able to make changes in the child's environment that will reduce the anxiety and distress experienced by the child. If parents can agree to strategies, the child may continue to enjoy consistent management across two households.

Keeping children informed is vital to their emotional wellbeing. They need to understand not only about the practical issues but also about the feelings that separation and divorce will arouse. These feelings will be similar to those encountered during bereavement and may include disbelief, denial, panic, anger, confusion, guilt, sadness, anxiety and depression. Ann Mitchell (1986) provides the following advice to parents coping with separation and divorce, which clinicians may find helpful:

- Explain why you and your spouse are separating and why the children will live with only one parent.
- Be aware that children might not share your feelings about the separation.
- Find someone else for your children to confide in at a time when you may be too upset to cope with your children's feelings yourself.
- Explain that divorce will end the marriage but not the parenting.
- Remember that children may behave differently at home and at school, and that it is often helpful for teachers to know about your separation.
- Make a positive effort to enable the child to keep in touch with the non-custodial parent.

Perhaps the most important feature is that the parents make every attempt to reassure the child that his relationship with each parent is maintained despite the separation/divorce.

Summary

We have described some of the problems that occur most frequently in the families we have seen, and there are no easy solutions to any of them. However, the recurring theme that has emerged is the need to keep an open dialogue between the parents and child, this it seems, is a crucial factor and should not be underestimated. There are no easy solutions to any of these problems and each family's requirements will be different. Therapists may need to consider that the role required of them is not to find the answer or provide a solution but rather to assist the family to use its own creativity and resources. Helping families to discover the skills they have provides the foundations for future growth.

Chapter 8 Direct Treatment of the Child

Direct fluency therapy

Indications for using direct fluency therapy

Following a course of indirect therapy focusing on parent–child interaction and any relevant family or child management issues, it may be necessary to undertake direct treatment of the child's fluency. This would be indicated by deterioration or an insufficient improvement in the child's speech, in spite of the changes that the parents have implemented and consolidated in their interaction and management. Direct therapy is also appropriate if a child has an excessively rapid rate of speaking which is not responding to the reduction in the parents' rate. Finally, there are children who may benefit from learning a strategy for overcoming specific initiation problems. Although relatively few preschool children have required direct therapy, in our experience for those who still have residual difficulties it has proved most successful.

Direct fluency therapy is always undertaken with the parents observing and participating in the activities in order to facilitate transfer into the home environment.

A cognitive behavioural approach

Speech modification techniques may be taught by use of two approaches:

- **Behavioural** methods whereby the clinician models the target behaviour, the child imitates and is positively reinforced when he achieves the desired effect. Homework and practice establishes the new pattern.
- **Cognitive** methods whereby the child understands the underlying concepts which are used to modify dysfluency, and is able to implement changes based on that awareness.

A combination of behavioural and cognitive methods has proved to be an effective approach with preschool children. We have found three main concepts to be central to fluency facilitation at this stage:

- Slow versus fast talking.
- Bumpy versus smooth talking.
- Hard versus easy talking.

In our experience most preschool children respond to reduction of rate as an effective speech modification technique. However, changing other aspects of speech production may be necessary if a child has specific unresolved struggle behaviours. It is important that any modification should maintain normal suprasegmental aspects of speech and should employ the least invasive of the techniques to establish fluency.

A cognitive approach helps the child to understand abstract concepts, such as slow/fast, bumpy/smooth, hard/easy. First, it is important to ensure that the child comprehends the meaning of each term in a concrete context. Therapy therefore begins with a series of activities which introduce these labels, for example, the slow versus fast concept may be taught by use of slow and fast trains or cars. This establishes the child's comprehension of the labels before they are used in a more abstract context.

Role of parents in direct therapy

Parents are actively involved in every stage of direct therapy sessions. The parents, clinician and child are seated together and participate equally in the activities which introduce the concepts for speech modification. Parents are instructed to imitate the clinician's mode of speech in order to provide an appropriate model for the child, i.e. if the therapy goal is rate reduction, the clinician and parents will be using a slower rate of speech throughout the session. Parents also participate in all activities which teach and reinforce the fluency rules. Homework activities are first practised within the therapy session and then carried out in the home setting.

Slow versus fast talking

Meyers and Woodford (1992) devised *The Fluency Development System for Young Children*, which teaches cognitively based fluency exercises. One of their three basic rules for facilitating fluency is: **use slow speech to talk more efficiently**. We have adapted their approach and the activities involved in order to help the dysfluent child learn to monitor his own rate and be able to slow down as appropriate. It may be necessary for the child to slow his rate at all times in order to achieve fluency. Alternatively, the child may adopt a slower rate only when he is being dysfluent.

The idea of slow versus fast is introduced in a play setting using cars, trains, dolls, or animals. The clinician first uses the slow/fast label with a series of different toys, thereby developing the child's understanding of the concept. This comprehension can be reinforced during sorting activities, e.g. fast animals versus slow animals. The child is then encouraged to verbalise the concept, describing the toys accordingly. When the clinician is satisfied that the child understands the fast versus slow concept, play characters are introduced which will adopt fast or slow speaking rates:

- Tortoise: a toy tortoise is used to depict slowness. The tortoise moves very slowly, and also talks slowly.
- Racehorse: a toy horse represents the fast concept. It gallops and races around and speaks at a very rapid rate.

These characters may be introduced by telling a story and using the toys to act it out. This is based on Aesop's fable of the Tortoise and the Hare. The tortoise and the racehorse decided to have a race, which the horse is convinced he will win. However, the horse races off so quickly his legs become all tangled and he falls down, whereas the tortoise proceeds at a sedate pace and wins the race. As the clinician recounts the story the contrasting rates of speech are used when describing either character.

The next step is to apply the fast/slow concept to the speaking process. The tortoise and racehorse start to talk. Tortoise speech is slow and stretched out but with normal volume, intonation and stress patterns. Racehorse speech is fast, jerky and almost unintelligible. The clinician models the two speaking styles and the child identifies which character is talking. An appropriate activity might be the tortoise and the racehorse saying which food they like. The clinician holds up a picture of a type of food and says *'I like apples'* using either the fast or slow rate. The child decides whether it was the tortoise or the racehorse talking and gives the picture to the appropriate character. When the child is reliably discriminating between the two speech styles, roles may be reversed. The child then attempts to use tortoise or racehorse speech and the clinician guesses which animal is talking. Further tortoise-talking activities should be introduced to reinforce a slow rate of speech at a simple linguistic level, e.g. picture naming — finding pictures hidden around the room; object naming — taking objects from a 'feeley bag'; lotto games; picture dominoes, etc. The child is then encouraged to play some games at home with his family, using tortoise speech. He is told that he must help his parents to learn tortoise speech, and that he should tell them if they are talking like a racehorse. Suitable games and activities are then demonstrated for practising tortoise speech at home, which the parents are instructed to carry out with the child. Parents may need reminding that the child is, however, only required to use tortoise talking during these activities.

Smooth versus bumpy talking

Smoothness is a quality which implies evenness, continuity and consistency, contrasting with bumpiness which is jerky, interrupted and irregular. Bumpy speech is characterised by breaks, blocks, repetitions and false starts, whereas smooth talking flows easily. Equipment should be prepared for concrete activities which will introduce the smooth versus bumpy concepts, comparing the physical texture of a variety of objects, e.g. shiny brown paper versus corrugated paper; smooth versus 'bubbled' plastic packing material; banana versus corn on the cob; leather purse versus beaded purse. When the child has understood the concept of smooth versus bumpy, the toy characters can be introduced:

- Snake: who glides slowly and smoothly along the ground.
- Frog: who jumps, stopping and starting.

The snake and frog may be used as characters in a story and their speech reflects the same features, i.e. the frog's talking is bu-bu-bumpy, whereas the snake flows the words smoothly. Identification activities teach the child to discriminate between the two speaking styles, deciding whether the snake or frog is speaking as previously described. The child then attempts 'snake speech' in a variety of tasks and games as above in the fast/slow section, and home practice is commenced once this has been established in the clinic.

Hard versus easy talking

This concept is most appropriate for a child who experiences difficulty initiating an utterance, especially if the speech is characterised by blocking. Such initiation problems may be effectively resolved using an easy onset approach, but this is a difficult concept to teach young children. The hard/easy contrast is best introduced with the more concrete notion of 'hardness' which is characterised by stiffness, becoming stuck or jammed, jerkiness and abrupt movement. The 'easy' concept is gentle, starting quietly and building up. Because the concepts are more specific, we usually introduce the toy characters at this stage:

- Soldier: a soldier is stiff — he stands and walks in a rigid, hard and jerky way and keeps getting his arms and legs stuck.
- Aeroplane: an aeroplane starts off completely still on the ground then

it slowly begins to move and gradually takes off until it is flying high in the air.

These toys can be played with to contrast their different styles. The child can role play being a soldier and an aeroplane. When the child has grasped the concepts using the toys, the notion of hard and easy talking can be introduced. Soldier speech is very jerky, loud and abrupt. Aeroplane speech starts gently and quietly then builds up. Therapy should consist of identification activities followed by expressive tasks previously described.

In our experience direct fluency therapy has been most effective in helping young dysfluent children overcome their difficulties. However, in certain cases children may not become completely fluent, but the amount and type of dysfluency changes: easy repetitions may replace prolongation and struggle behaviour. We have found that these children often have strong neurological and linguistic factors which are affecting their fluency. They may continue to require therapy support as they grow older, but this input in the initial stages will have reduced the effect of the dysfluency on their early social and emotional development.

Language therapy for the dysfluent child

Co-occurrence of both language and fluency problems in preschool children may arise when:

- A child who has been receiving speech and language therapy for language problems begins to manifest dysfluent behaviours. This may be a delayed period of normal non-fluency or could also be the effect of an overload in the linguistic demands placed on a child's system. In either case it should be managed with care in order to prevent the development of a stutter.
- A child who is referred for dysfluency but assessment reveals underlying linguistic difficulties, for example, specific word-finding problems. A dysfluency problem may mask an underlying language deficit, distracting parents or a clinician from investigating the child's linguistic abilities.

A child who is manifesting both language difficulties and dysfluency is especially disadvantaged and requires careful management. As we have discussed (Chapter 5) impoverished language or specific language difficulties may make a significant contribution to a child's dysfluency. However, attending to the child's linguistic performance is likely to increase pressure on the child and result in a deterioration of the fluency. It is therefore essential that treatment is directed at providing the child with the necessary linguistic capacities but without placing too many demands on his fluency.

Language therapy should therefore be focused upon developing the child's receptive linguistic abilities with minimal emphasis on actual output. Hence, for a child with an impoverished vocabulary, treatment should aim to increase his comprehension of a wide range of lexical items without requiring him to practise using the vocabulary expressively. Similarly, syntactic structures and word order can be taught at a receptive level, thus developing the child's competence without placing undue pressure on performance. The assumption being that the child will begin to use these newly acquired structures only when he is ready to do so spontaneously.

Case Example

Matthew, aged 3;9, was referred for management of his dysfluency. Assessment revealed that 18% of his speech was dysfluent, featuring part-word repetitions and prolongations. His rate of speech was 139 words spoken per minute. His comprehension was at a three information-carrying word level and his BPVS scores were as follows: 90 standard score, 26th percentile, 2;11 age equivalent. His expressive output was restricted to simple sentence structures with syntactic immaturities. On the WFVS he scored at a 3-year level. There was evidence of a word-finding difficulty, marked by overuse of deixis and some use of description of an item, e.g. in the water, mans in it, in the, it a (boat). Assessment of the parent–child interaction indicated that both parents were over-directive during play, controlling the activity using lots of imperatives. They also used lots of questions and spoke rapidly. Six weeks of interaction therapy targeted these areas and both parents adopted a less directive style, using more commenting and reducing their speech rate. As a result of this Matthew became more verbal during play and began to expand his lexicon. Matthew's language skills improved and his dysfluency reduced in amount and featured whole-word and part-word repetitions.

Phonological therapy for the dysfluent child

If a preschool child presents with both dysfluency and phonological impairment it is, once again, important to acknowledge the interaction between these problems. If a child has difficulty in selecting and/or producing the correct phoneme in order to achieve intelligibility, this may affect fluency levels. Treatment of the phonological system may result in increased dysfluency as the child becomes more aware of the physical act of speaking. Attempts to modify 'incorrectly' produced phonemes may increase emotional pressure on the child and adversely affect fluency. Phonological therapy should therefore target the child's listening/discrimination skills, with no emphasis on changes in production. Metaphon therapy (Howell and Dean, 1991) provides a useful framework for such an approach. Furthermore, parents should be instructed not to correct the child's speech production, but to provide a clear model, e.g. if the child says 'tup' the parents says '*Yes it's a* **c** *up*'.

The parent should not say *'not tup, cup. You say cup'*. This emphasis on developing the child's awareness of the target model will not jeopardise his fluency, as there is no direct focus on changing the child's production of speech.

Some authorities advocate the use of oral motor exercises or 'drilling' to improve a child's physical competence and coordination for speech. They recommend that a child practises speech sound production at the individual phoneme level, in order to enhance intelligibility of speech at the word and sentence level. This approach may be appropriate for a child whose speech is affected by a specific motor deficit, e.g. dyspraxia, dysarthria. However, we would be concerned that any emphasis on the production of phonemes would result in increased pressure on the child's limited capacities and result in fluency breakdown. Furthermore, as soon as the phoneme was introduced at a word level, the linguistic dimension would place greater demands on the child's system.

Case Example

Gary, aged 4;4, was referred for assessment and treatment of his dysfluency. His case had been monitored by his local speech therapy service for 18 months as he also had moderately delayed phonological development. Gary's parents were publicans and they lived on site. His father stuttered severely, as did his grandfather, and his mother had a hearing loss and spoke very loudly and rapidly. Gary also had a sister who was 8 years old. Speech and language assessments revealed Gary's sophisticated linguistic ability: his receptive vocabulary yielded a standard score of 126 and his naming vocabulary was at a $6\frac{1}{2}$ year level. However, his connected speech was almost completely unintelligible. Phonological analysis revealed consistent patterns of fronting velar plosives, stopping of alveolar and palatal fricatives and cluster reduction. Gary's articulatory rate was rapid: 136 fluent words spoken per minute. His dysfluency was characterised by part-word repetitions and prolongations, calculated at 12% dysfluency. Six interaction therapy sessions were undertaken aimed at reducing parental directiveness and rate reduction. During each session Gary also did some discrimination tasks focusing on the front/back phonological process. Further listening exercises were set for homework and the parents were instructed not to correct Gary's speech. During the consolidation period Gary's parents reported that his fluency increased significantly although his intelligibility remained poor. The family attended three review appointments at 12-week intervals, during which interaction styles were monitored and further listening exercises set. During this period Gary became highly fluent and his phonological difficulties began to resolve. Two years later Gary remains fluent and his speech is completely intelligible.

Summary

We have described methods of directly treating the dysfluent child. Direct fluency therapy, aimed at providing the child with fluency enhancing strategies, is advocated for a child whose dysfluency remains unresolved following a period of interaction therapy. Therapists should be aware that many children show improvements in their language and phonological skills as a result of interaction therapy. We have found it helpful to wait until the consolidation period has been completed before making the decision to work directly on fluency or speech and language skills, as change continues to occur during this period. Treatment of a dysfluent child's language or phonological skills has also been outlined, with a particular emphasis on building a child's competence without any demands being placed on his performance.

Appendix I

CHILD ASSESSMENT

Name: .... Date of birth: ....

Age: .... Clinician: ....

GENERAL BEHAVIOUR

SEPARATION

CO-OPERATION

MANNER

ANXIETY/TENSION

ATTENTION

FIDGETING

COGNITIVE SKILLS

ORGANISATIONAL SKILLS

DRAWING

PLAY

VERBAL COMPREHENSION

(a) OBJECT MATERIAL

TWO WORD LEVEL

(i) Equipment: brick, spoon, doll, knife, box, plate and cup

Put the knife in the cup ______________________

Put the brick on the plate ______________________

Put the doll in the box ______________________

(ii) NEGATION

Equipment: 2 dolls & spoon (place next to one doll)

which doll has no spoon ______________________

Equipment: 2 dolls: 1 seated & 1 lying

which doll is not sitting ______________________

(iii) DESCRIPTION

Equipment: Dirty & clean doll

Show me the dirty doll ______________________

Equipment: Wet & dry doll's dress

Show me the wet dress ______________________

(iv) SIZE

Equipment: Big & little spoon, big & little cup

Show me the big spoon ______________________

Show me the little cup ______________________

THREE WORD LEVEL

Equipment: brick, spoon, doll, knife, box, plate & cup.

Put the knife under the plate ______________________

Put the brick in the cup______________________

Put the spoon under the box ______________________

Give me the plate & spoon ______________________

FOUR WORD LEVEL

Equipment: as above + pencil

Put the spoon & the knife on the plate ______________________

Put the pencil in the box& the knife in the cup ______________________

Put the brick under the box & give me the plate

____

Give me the cup, the brick & the doll

____

(b) <u>PICTURE MATERIAL</u>

<u>Equipment:</u> Pictures

(i) who isn't sleeping ______
(ii) who is brushing his hair ______
tell me about this one ______
(iii) who has got lots of bricks ______
tell me about this one ______
(iv) who is going to drink the juice ______
tell me about this one ______
(v) who has washed her face ______
(vi) which one am I talking about:
he's playing with a doll ______
she's playing with the car ______

<u>COMPREHENSION WITHOUT VISUAL CLUES</u>

COMMANDS

Open the door & switch on the light ______
Stand up & clap your hands ______

QUESTIONS

Why do you brush your hair ______

How did you get here today ______
Where do tigers live ______

CAUSE & EFFECT

What would happen if a wheel fell off a bike ______
What would you do if a boy hit you ______

DEFINITIONS

Tell me what ..... means or Tell me what a... is

1. hat. chocolate ______
2. running. washing ______
3. sticky. hungry ______
4. funny. scared ______
5. disappear. float ______

WORD LISTS

Tell me as many animals as you can in one minute

______

______

COMPREHENSION SUMMARY

Length of utterance
Syntactic complexity
Semantic complexity
BPVS score:

EXPRESSIVE LANGUAGE

Renfrew WFVS: Age equivalent
Comments

Linguistic analysis
form
content
use

Word finding ability

PHONOLOGY

- intelligibility
- delayed/deviant pattern

PROSODY
- volume
- intonation
- voice quality

SOCIAL SKILLS

Observation & eye contact

Listening skills

Turn taking

Position

Facial expression

Gesture

DYSFLUENCY

1. **Type**

WWR	number of repetitions
PWR	number of repetitions
	schwa
Prolongations	length of prolongation
Struggle	
Other	

2. **Locus** of dysfluency in: sentence
   word
   syllable

3. **Percentage of dysfluency**

$$\frac{DW}{TWS} \times 100 = \%DW$$

4. **Articulatory rate**

$$\frac{FWS}{Fsecs} \times 60 = FWS/M$$

5. **Actual rate**

$$\frac{WS}{Tsecs} \times 60 = WS/M$$

6. **Occurrence in pragmatic categories**

initiation	request	response
interruption	comment	interrupted utterance
imperative		

7. **Concomitant facial/body movements**

8. **Avoidance**

9. **Awareness**

CHILD INTERVIEW

Nursery/School

Attitude

Teachers

Friends

What do you do?

What do you like doing?

What don't you like doing?

Teasing Fights

Home/Family

Relationship with siblings/parents

What do you like doing?

What don't you like doing?

Speech

Why here?

How are you getting on with your talking?

Is it sometimes difficult to talk What happens?

It is sometimes easy to talk. When?

When did it start getting hard?

Can you help yourself?

Do you want help?

How would life be different if no dysfluency?

Anyone else in family same difficulty?

Best thing that ever happened to you:

Worst thing that ever happened to you:

What do you do when you have problem:

One change about you:

TRANSCRIPTION OF DYSFLUENCY

NAME: ______________________________ **DATE:** __________

CLINICIAN: ______________________________

Number of dysfluent words	**(DW)..................**			
Total number of words spoken	**(TWS)................**			
Total time in seconds	**(Tsec).................**			
Number of fluent words	**(FW)..................**			
Time of fluent speech	**(Fsec)................**			
Percentage of dysfluency:	=	$\frac{DW}{TWS}$ x 100	=	..................%DW
Articulatory rate:	=	$\frac{FWS}{Fsec}$ x 60	=	..................FWS/M
Actual rate:	=	$\frac{TWS}{Tsec}$ x 60	=	..................WS/M

INTERACTION PROFILE

NON VERBAL		VERBAL
	Directiveness	
	Following child's lead	
		Turn taking
Listening		Balance of conversation
		Interrupting
	Giving time to respond	
	Pausing	
		Rate
Gaining child's attention		
		Intelligibility
Observation		Volume
Eye contact with child		Fluency
Shared focus of attention		Prosody
Facial expression		Complexity: syntactic
Animation		semantic
Intrigue		Semantic contingency
Touch		
Gesture		Initiation- questions/requests
		- imperatives
Position		- comments
- level		- other
- mobility		
- orientation		Commenting
- proximity		Responding
		Repetition
Manner		Rephrasing
- warmth		Maintaining topic
- attachment	Reinforcement	Repair
	Conflict management	
	Choice of activity	
	Response to dysfluency	

Appendix II

Picture material

1.

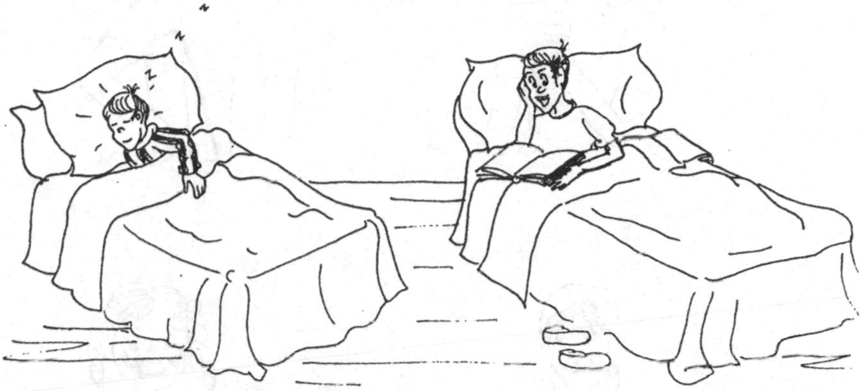

2.

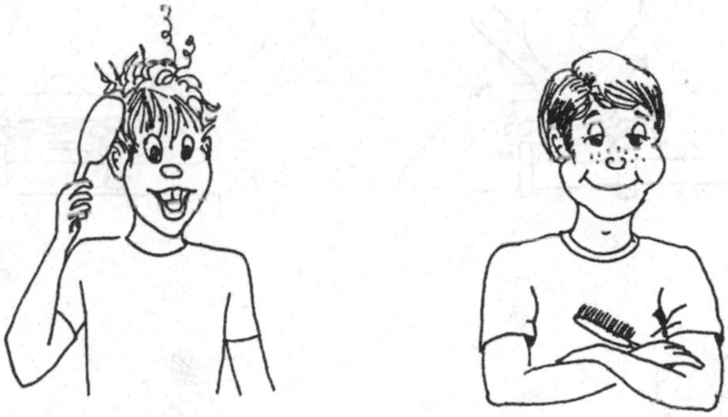

3.

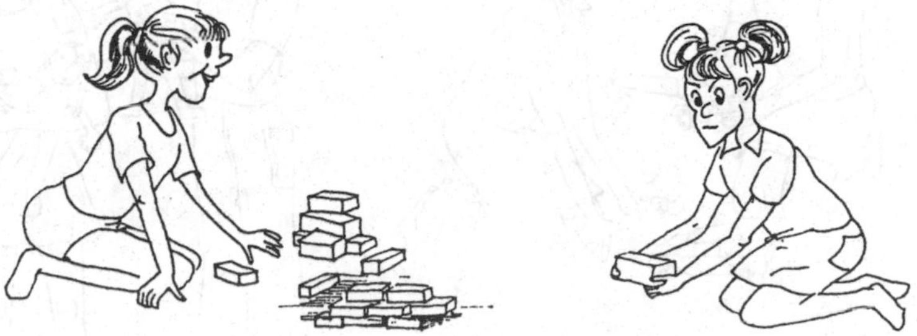

4.

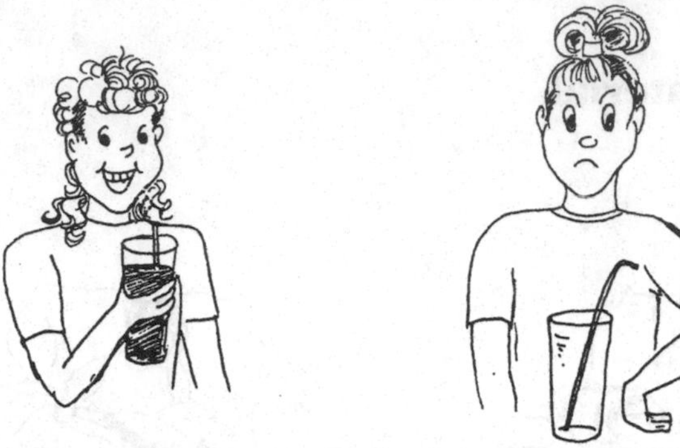

5.

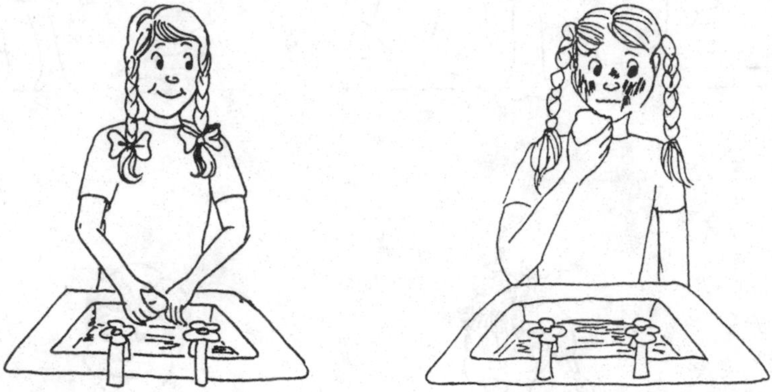

6.

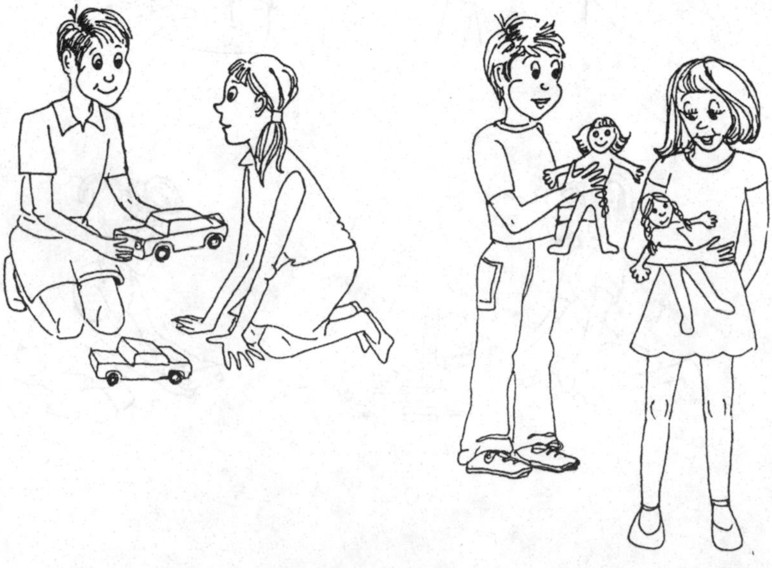

Appendix III

Parent Interview

Child

Family name: ....

First name(s): ....

Sex: .... Date of birth: .... Age on date of interview ....

School/Nursery: ....

Home address:..

....

....

Post Code: .... Tel: ....

Mother	**Father**
Family name:	Family name: ....
First name(s) :	First name (s) ....
Date of birth:	Date of birth : ....

Address, if different from child's address: ....

....

Post code: .... Tel :...

Referred by : .... Date of referral: ....

GP name: .... Address: ....

....

Child's first Language: ....

Languages used in the home: ....

Interviewer: .... Date : ....

PRESENTING PROBLEM

What is the problem?

Does the child have any other problems apart from the dysfluency?

Which problem would you like to deal with first?

Describe the dysfluency in detail

Date of onset Gradual/Sudden

Any major events at this time?

How did it develop?

What do you think caused the dysfluency?

Frequency? Severity?

Are there periods of fluency?

Context: When is the dysfluency worse?

When is the child more fluent?

Do you refer to the problem?

How do you refer to it?

What do you do or say when your child is dysfluent?

Mother:

Father:

Other members of family:

How does the dysfluency affect the family?

How does the dysfluency make you feel?

Mother:

Father:

Previous therapy:

Expectations of therapy:

GENERAL HEALTH

How is the child's general health?

Allergies/asthma/eczema

Headaches Stomach aches:

Childhood illnesses: Fits/faints
Convulsions

Medication

Hospitalisations in patient:

Accidents

Out patient

Hearing test eye test

Attendances at other clinics including child guidance

Overactive or restless? Stay still if expected to? Fidgety?

Concentration? Longest time on something interesting?

Clumsiness? Preferred hand and foot?

Twitches/eye blinking, head banging

BEHAVIOUR

<u>Eating</u>

Difficulties: Fussy:

Feed self:

<u>Sleeping</u>

Bedtime: When wakes:

Sleep through the night: Stay in own bed:

Daytime sleep:

Talking in sleep/Sleepwalking: Nightmares:

Toilet training

When dry by day: By night:

Problems:

Enuresis: Soiling: Constipation:

COMMUNICATION

How does child communicate? (include non-verbal)

Does the child understand you?

Do you understand the child?

Do others understand the child?

Any difficulties with pronunciation?

Do you speak for the child?

Do others speak for the child?

Speak as well as others of same age?

Spontaneity of talking?

PERSONALITY

What sort of child is he:

Happy/miserable Cry

Worry Irritable Sulky

Temper tantrums and situations:

Fears Fussy Routines/Rituals

Comfort habits (sucking thumb, blanket, nail biting, soft toy, dummy)

Separation difficulties:

Tears on going to nursery/school

Nursery/school refusal

Reaction to new people Shy/Clinging

Reaction to new places

RELATIONSHIP WITH PEERS

How does the child get on with other children?

Friends? See them outside nursery/school?

Prefers children of own age? Younger or older?

Girls or boys? Leader or follower?

Bully? Bullied? Fights?

Teased? Member of club/group?

RELATIONSHIP WITH SIBLINGS

Position in the family?

Names and ages of siblings

How do they get on? Do they play together?

Particularly attached to any siblings? How is this shown?

Squabbling? Who with?

Come to blows? Jealousy?

Do the siblings have any particular problems?

RELATIONSHIP WITH ADULTS

	Mother's reply	Father's reply
How does the child get on with:		
Which child in the family do you relate to more easily?		
How is affection shown?		
Is the child easy to get on with?		
Who does the child take after?		
What do you like about your child?		
What aspects do you find difficult?		

How does the child get on with other adults? With nursery staff/teachers?

SEX EDUCATION

Interest in opposite sex?

Instructed in sex?

Questions asked?
How do parents respond?

Masturbation?

SCHOOLING

	When/How often	Reaction/Progress
Mother/toddler group		
Playgroup		
Nursery/type		
School/type		

Are any changes planned?

Do parents see staff?

Feedback from staff

Progress: Reading? Writing? Numeracy?

FAMILY STRUCTURE AND HISTORY

How long married/together?

Have you had any separations? (circumstances)

Previous long-term relationships/marriages?

Children?

Mother had any miscarriages, still births, terminations? (circumstances)

Children adopted or fostered?

PERSONAL BACKGROUND	MOTHER	FATHER
Place of birth/age		
Religion		
Occupation		
Education		
Description of Personality		
General health/illness		
Medication		
Depression? Suicide attempt?		
Have you seen a counsellor for any reason?		
Seen by psychiatrist?		
Stuttering		
Difficulty learning to speak/read/write/spell		
Alcohol related problems		
Drug related problems		
Epilepsy		
Court appearances		

PARENT FAMILY BACKGROUND

MOTHER'S PARENTS	GRANDMOTHER	GRANDFATHER
Age		
Health		
Where they live		
Relationship with child		
Occupation		
Marital state		
Siblings/place in family		
Upbringing		
Date and cause of death		
Reaction and management of bereavement		

FATHER'S PARENTS	GRANDMOTHER	GRANDFATHER
Age		
Health		
Where they live		
Relationship with child		
Occupation		
Marital state		
Siblings/place in family		
Upbringing		
Date and cause of death		
Reaction and management of bereavement		

EXTENDED FAMILY HISTORY

Brothers, sisters, aunts, uncles, nieces, nephews	Mother's family	Father's family
Stuttering		
Psychiatric treatment		
Depression		
Suicide/attempt		
Difficulty learning to speak/read/write/spell		
Drug related problems		
Alcohol related problems		
Epilepsy/other medical		
Court appearances		

HOME CIRCUMSTANCES

House or flat? Own/rented/council Number of bedrooms?

Sleeping arrangements?

Others in home?

Child care arrangements

Place to play? Inside Outside

How long lived in the neighbourhood? Do you like it?

Any financial difficulties?

Income support

Maintenanance

FAMILY LIFE AND RELATIONSHIPS

Parental Relationship

How do you two get on?

Things enjoyed doing together?

How spend evenings and weekends?

Do you spend time together on your own?

Allocation of child care and household tasks?

Do you have friends?

How do you resolve problems in the family?

Single Parents

Contact with other parent:

Relationship with other parent:

How did you separate?

How did it affect child?

Problems with custody?

Any other relationships at present:

How long alone:

Support network:

Parent–child activities

What toys or activities does child enjoy?

Go out together?

Play together? Help make things?

Does child need help with dressing? Who helps?

Who takes to nursery/school?

Does the child help with washing up, tidying, errands etc?

Mother or Father's child

Confide in father?:

mother?:

Attachment to other adults?

ANTI-SOCIAL BEHAVIOUR AND DISCIPLINE

Naughty/Disobedient? Destructive?

Fire setting? Lies?

Stealing?

Truanting from school? Run away from home?

Allowed to climb on furniture? Allowed to leave house without saying where he is going?

Restrictions on friends: TV:

Any other family rules:

What do you do if child is naughty?

How does child react?

Are you consistent?

Pocket money? How much?

CHILD'S DEVELOPMENTAL HISTORY

Pregnancy

Mother's health during pregnancy?

Home or hospital delivery? Complications?

Maturity? Birth weight?

Mother's health after pregnancy?

Was this pregnancy planned?

How did child's birth affect the family?

Development in infancy

Difficulties breathing or sucking?

Convulsions? Jaundice?

Breast or bottle fed? Weaning when? Introduction of solids?

Placid or active? Crying? Response to mother?

Sitting unsupported? Walking?

First words with meaning? First simple sentences?

Comparison with siblings?

Any developmental problems?

SEPARATIONS

Ever away from home without parents? (holidays, hospitals, etc)

How looked after?

Reaction?

EMOTIONAL EXPRESSION/SENSITIVITY

How does he express feelings?

How does the child respond if a person or animal is hurt?

How does the child react if something goes wrong?

Would you describe your child as sensitive?

How would your child's life be different if he wasn't dysfluent?

How would your life be different if he wasn't dysfluent?

Note future impending changes for child or family

SUMMARY OF ISSUES

MANAGEMENT

Appendix IV

The summary chart

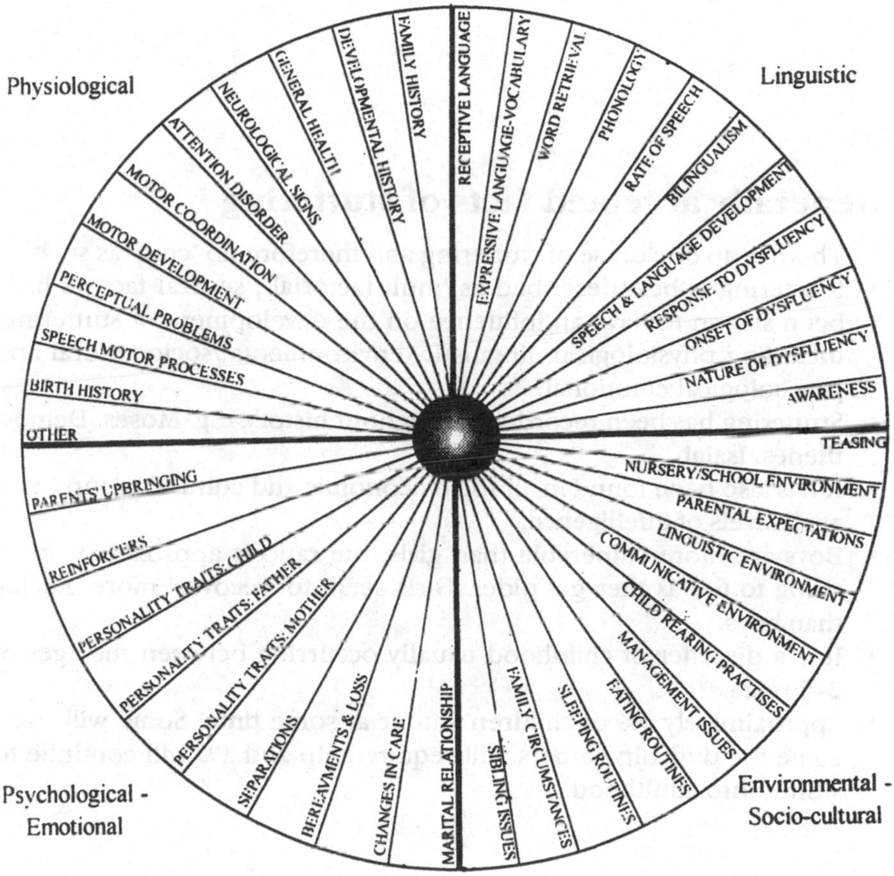

Appendix V

Generally accepted facts of stuttering

- There is no *one* cause of stuttering and therefore no 'cure' as such.
- Stuttering is best described as 'multifactorial'; several factors have been shown to have an influence on the development of stuttering, including physiological, linguistic, environmental/sociocultural and psychological/emotional.
- Stuttering has been recorded throughout history, e.g. Moses, Demosthenes, Isaiah.
- It has also been found in all socio-economic and cultural groups, and at all levels of intelligence.
- Boys are more vulnerable than girls, the ratio is approximately 3:1 rising to 6:1 as they get older. Girls seem to 'recover' more quickly than boys.
- It is a disorder of childhood usually occurring between the ages of 2–5 years.
- Approximately 5% of children stutter at some time. Some will overcome the difficulty; others will require help and 1% will continue to stutter into adulthood.

Appendix VI

SPECIAL TIME - INSTRUCTION SHEET

Special Time lasts for five minutes only and should not be extended.

Allow your child to select an activity, toy or game of his choice. This should not be reading a book, watching television or playing a lively outdoor game. When the child has chosen what to do, go to a room where you will not be disturbed and deal with any obvious distractions eg T.V., radio. Play with your child, focusing your attention on him/her and <u>what</u> he or she is saying (not how he or she is saying it). When the allotted time has finished record your Special Time on the task sheet, writing what you did and how you felt about it.

Appendix VII

5 MINUTES SPECIAL TIME TASK SHEET

PARENT'S NAME.................................. CHILD'S NAME..................................

ADDRESS ....

TARGETS FOR SPECIAL TIME ....

DATE	DESCRIPTION OF ACTIVITY	COMMENTS OR FEELINGS

Example of completed task sheet

SPECIAL TIME TASK SHEET

Parent's name: .... Child's name: ....

Target for Special Time: ....

Date	Description of activity	Comments or feelings
4.6.94	We played with the Duplo We made a house with a garage	Josh is very good at building and I enjoyed it too. Almost forgot to stop after 5 minutes. Josh did not protest today

References

Accordi, M., Bianchi, R., Consolaro, C., Tronchin, F., De Filippi, R., Pasqualon, L., Ugo, E. and Croalto, L. (1983) L'Eziopatogensi della balnuzie: Studio statistico su 2802 casi. *Acta Phoniatrica Latino* **5**, 171–180.

Adams, M., Freeman, F. and Conture, E. (1985) Laryngeal dynamics of stutterers. In: Curlee, R.F. and Perkins, R.H. (eds). *Nature and Treatment of Stuttering: New Directions*. San Diego: College Hill Press.

Adler, J.B. and Starkweather, C.W. (1979) Oral and laryngeal reaction times in stutterers. *ASHA* **21**, 769 (abstract).

Andrews, J. and Andrews, M. (1990) *Family Based Treatment in Communicative Disorders: A Systematic Approach*. Dekalb, IL: Janelle Publications.

Andrews, G. and Harris, M. (1964) The syndrome of stuttering, *Clinics in Developmental Medicine*, No. 7. London: Spastics Society Medical Education and Information Unit in association with Heinemann Medical Books.

Andrews, G., Craig, A., Feyer, A.N., Hodinott, S., Howie, P. and Neilson, M. (1983) Stuttering: a review of research findings and theories circa 1982. *Journal of Speech and Hearing Disorders* **48**, 226–246.

Andronico, M. and Blake, I. (1971) The application of filial therapy to young childen with stuttering problems. *Journal of Speech and Hearing Disorders* **36**, 377–381.

Argyle, M. (1975) *Bodily Communication*. London: Methuen.

Armson, J. and Kalinowski, J. (1994) Interpreting results of the fluent speech paradigm in stuttering research: difficulties in separating cause from effect. *Journal of Speech and Hearing Research* **37**, 69–82.

Bell, and Harper, (1977) *Child Effects on Adults*. Hillsdown, NJ: Lawrence Erlbaum.

Bernstein-Ratner, N. and Sih, C.C. (1987) Effects of gradual increases in sentences length and complexity on children's dysfluency. *Journal of Speech and Hearing Research* **52**, 278–287.

Bloch, E.L. and Goodstein, L.D. (1971) Functional speech disorders and personality: a decade of research. *Journal of Speech and Hearing Disorders* **36**, 295–314.

Blood, G.W. and Scider, R. (1981) The concomitant problems of young stutterers. *Journal of Speech and Hearing Disorders* **46**, 31–33.

Bloodstein, O. (1987) *A Handbook on Stuttering*. Chicago: National Easter Seal Society.

Bloodstein, O. (1993) *Stuttering: The Search for a Cause and Cure.* Chicago: Allyn & Bacon.

Bloodstein, O. (1995) *A Handbook on Stuttering*. San Diego: Singular Publishing Group.

Branden, N. (1972) The Disowned Self. New York: Bantain Books.

Broen, P. (1972) The verbal environment of the language learning child. *ASHA* monographs, No. 17. American Speech Language Hearing Association.

Boberg, E., Yendall, L., Schoptlocher, D. and Bo-lassen, P. (1983) The effects of an intensive behavioural programme on the distribution of EEG alpha power in stutterers during the processing of verbal and visuo spatial information. *Journal of Fluency Disorders* **8**, 245–263.

Christensen, A., Phillips. S., Glasgow, R.E. and Johnson S.M. (1983) Parental characteristics and interactional dysfunction in families with child behaviour problems: a preliminary investigation. *Journal of Abnormal Child Psychology* **11**(1), 153–166.

Conture, E. (1990) *Stuttering* (second edition). Englewood Cliffs, NJ: Prentice Hall.

Conture, E.G. (1982) *Stuttering*. Englewood Cliffs, NJ: Prentice Hall.

Conture, E.G. and Caruso, A.J. (1987) Assessment and diagnosis of childhood dysfluency. In: Rustin, L., Purser, H. and Rowley, D. (eds). *Progress in the Treatment of Fluency Disorders*. London: Taylor & Francis.

Conture, E.G. and Kelly, E. (1991) Young stutterers' non speech behaviours during stuttering. *Journal of Speech and Hearing Research* **34**, 1041–1056.

Cooper, E.B. (1987) The Cooper personalized fluency control therapy. In: Rustin, L., Purser, H. and Rowley, D. (eds). *Progress in the Treatment of Fluency Disorders*. London: Taylor & Francis.

Cox, N.J., Seider, R.A. and Kidd, K.K. (1984) Some environmental factors and hypotheses for stuttering in families with several stutterers. *Journal of Speech and Hearing Research* **27**, 543–548.

Crystal, D. (1987) Towards a 'bucket' theory of language disability: taking account of interaction between linguistic levels. *Clinical Linguistics and Phonetics* **1**, 7–22.

Cullinan, W.L. and Springer, M.T. (1980) Voice initiation times in stuttering and non stuttering children. *Journal of Speech and Hearing Research* **23**, 344–360.

Dalton, P. and Hardcastle, W.J. (1977) *Disorders of Fluency*. New York: Elsevier.

D'Ardenne, P. and Mahtani, A. (1989) *Transcultural Therapy in Action*. London: Sage.

Davis, S. and Aslam, M. (1981) Eastern treatment for Eastern health? In: Cheetham, J., James, W., Loney, M., Mayor, B. and Prescott, W. *Social and Community Work in a Multi-Racial Society*. London: Harper and Row.

De Joy, D. and Gregory, H. (1985) The relationship between age and frequency of disfluency in preschool children. *Journal of Fluency Disorders* **10**, 107–122.

De Shazer, S. (1982) Some conceptual distinctions are more useful than others. Family Process **21**, 71–84.

Dunn, L.M. and Dunn, L.M. (1981) *Peabody Picture Vocabulary Test — Revised*. Circle Pines, MN: American Guidance Service.

Dunn, L.M., Dunn, L.M. and Whetton, C. with Pintilie, D. (1982) *British Picture Vocabulary Scale*. Windsor: NFER-Nelson.

Dyregrov, A. (1990) (reprinted 1992). *Grief in Children: A Handbook for Adults*. London: Jessica Kingsley.

Faber, A. and Mazlish, E. (1980) *How to Talk So Kids Will Listen and Listen So Kids Will Talk*. New York: Avon Books.

Falloon, I.R.H. (1988) *Handbook of Behavioural Family Therapy*. London: The Guildford Press.

Farber, S. (1981) *Identical Twins Reared Apart: A Reanalysis*. New York: Basic Books.

Gaines, N., Runyan, C., Meyers, S. (1991) A comparison of young stutters' fluent versus stuttered utterances on measures of length and complexity. *Journal of Speech and Hearing Research* **34**, 37–42.

Ginott, H. (1969) *Between Parent and Child*. New York: Avon Books.

Goodenough, . (1982) *DRAW-A-MAN TEST*. Cambridge: LDA Living and Learning.

German, D.J. (1989) *Test of Word Finding*. Leicester: Taskmaster.

Girolametto, L.E. (1988) Developing dialogue skills 'the effects of a conversational model of language intervention'. In: Marfo, K. (Ed.). *Parent–Child Interaction and Developmental Disabilities*. New York: Praeger.

Glasner, P. (1970) Developmental view. In: Sheehan, J. (Ed.). *Stuttering Research and Therapy*. New York: Harper and Row.

Gregory, H. (1986) Environmental manipulation and family counselling. In: Shames, G. and Rubin, H. (eds). *Stuttering: Then and Now*. Columbus: Charles E. Merrill.

Gregory, H.H. (1985) Prevention of stuttering: management of early stages. In: Curlee, R.F. and Perkins, W.H. (eds). *Nature and Treatment of Stuttering: New Directions*. New York: Taylor & Francis.

Gregory, H.H. and Hill, D. (1984) Stuttering therapy for children. In W.H. Perkins (Ed.) *Current Therapy of Communication Disorders: Stuttering Disorders*. New York: Thieme-Stratton.

Grunwell, P. (1985) Some conceptual distinctions are more useful than others. *Family Process* **21**, 71–84.

Haynes, W. and Hood, S. (1978) Dysfluency changes in children as a function of the systematic modification of linguistic complexity. *Journal of Community Disorders* **11**, 79–93.

Heyhow, R. and Levy, C. (1989) *Working with Stuttering: A Personal Construct Approach*. Oxon: Winslow Press.

Holme, T. and Rahe, R. (1967) Social Adjustment Rating Scale. *Journal of Psychosomatic Research* **11**, 213–218.

Howell, J. and Dean, E. (1991) *Treating Phonological Disorders in Children: Metaphon — Theory to Practice*. Kibworth: Far Communications.

Howell, P. and Vause, L. (1986) Acoustic analysis and perception of vowels in stuttered speech. *Journal of the Acoustical Society of America* **79**, 1571–1579.

Howell, P. and Williams, M. (1992) Acoustic analysis and perception of vowels in children's and teenager's stuttered speech. *Journal of the Accoustical Society of America* **91**, 1697–1706.

Howie, P.M. (1981) Concordance for stuttering in monozygothic and dizygotic twin pairs. *Journal of Speech and Hearing Research* **24**, 317–321.

Johnson, W. (1959) *The Onset of Stuttering*. Minneapolis: University of Minnesota Press.

Kasprisin-Burrelli A., Egolf, D. and Shames, G. (1972) A comparison of parental verbal behaviour with stuttering and non stuttering children. *Journal of Communication Disorders* **5**, 335–346.

Kelman, E. and Schneider, C. (1994) Parent–child interaction: an alternative approach to the management of children's language difficulties. *Child Language Teaching and Therapy* **10**(1).

Kidd, K.K. (1977) A genetic perspective on stuttering. *Journal of Fluency Disorders* **2**, 259–269.

Kidd, K. (1983) Recent progress on the genetics of stuttering. In: Ludlow, C. and Cooper, C. (eds). *Genetic Aspects of Speech and Language*. New York: Academic Press.

Kidd, K.K. (1984) Stuttering as a genetic disorder. In: Curlee, R.F. and Perkins, R.H. (eds). *Nature and Treatment of Stuttering: New Directions*. San Diego: College Hill Press.

Kidd, K.K., Kidd J.R. and Records, M.A. (1978) The possible causes of the sex ratio in stuttering and its implications. *Journal of Fluency Disorders* 3, 13–23.

Kline, M. and Starkweather, C. (1979) Receptive and expressive language performance in young stutterers. *ASHA* 21, 797 (Abstract).

Kubler-Ross, E. (1969) *On Death and Dying*. London: Tavistock.

LDA (1988) *What's Wrong Cards*. Cambridge: Living and Learning.

Lamb, M.E. and Easterbrooks, M.A. (1981) Individual differences in parental sensitivity: origins, components and consequences. In: Lamb, M.E. and Sherrod, L.R. (eds). *Infant Social Cognition: Empirical and Theoretical Considerations*. Hillsdale, NJ: Erlbaum.

Langlois, A., Hanrahan, L. and Inouye (1986) A comparison of interactions between stuttering children, non-stuttering children and their mothers. *Journal of Fluency Disorders* 11, 263–273.

Lasalle, L. and Conture, E. (1991)Eye contact between young stutterers and their mothers. *Journal of Fluency Disorders* 16, 173–199.

Lees, R. (1994) Of what value is a measure of the stutterer's fluency? *Folia Phoniatrica et Logopaedica* 46, 223–231.

Logan, K. and Conture, E. (1995) Length, grammatical complexity and rate differences in stuttered and fluent conversational utterances of children who stutter. *Journal of Fluency Disorders* 20(1), 35–61.

Lytton, H. and Zwirner, W. (1975) Compliance and its controlling stimuli observed in a natural setting. *Developmental Psychology* 15, 256–268.

Masidlover, M. and Knowles, W. (1982) *Detailed Test of Comprehension: Derbyshire Language Scheme*. Derbyshire County Council.

Merits-Patterson, R. and Reed C. (1981) Disfluencies in the speech of language disordered children. *Journal of Speech and Hearing Research* 46, 55–56.

Meyers, S.C. (1991). Interactions with pre-operational pre-school stutterers: how will this influency therapy? In: Rustin, L. *Parents, Families and the Stuttering Child*. Kibworth: Far Communications.

Meyers, S. and Freeman, F. (1985a) Are mothers of stutterers different? An investigation of social communicative interactions. *Journal of Fluency Disorders* 10, 193–209.

Meyers, S. and Freeman, S. (1985b) Interruptions as a variable in stuttering and disfluency. *Journal of Speech and Hearing Research* 28, 428–435.

Meyers S. and Freeman, F. (1985c) Mother and child speech rates as a variable in stuttering and disfluency. *Journal of Speech and Hearing Research* 28, 436–444.

Meyers S.C. and Woodford, L.L. (1992) *The Fluency Development System for Young Children*. Buffalo, NY: United Educational Services Inc.

Miller, W.H. (1975) Systematic Parent Training: Procedures, Cases and Issues. Champaign, IL: Research Press.

Minuchin, S. (1974) *Families and Family Therapy*. Boston, MA: Harvard University Press.

Mitchell, A. (1986) *Coping with Separation and Divorce*. Edinburgh: Chambers.

Moore, M. and Nystul, M. (1979) Parent child attitudes and communication processes in families with stutterers and families with nonstutterers. *British Journal of Disorders of Communication* 14(3), 174–179.

Moore, W.H. Jr (1984) Hemispheric Alpha assynmetries during an electromyographic biofeedback procedure for stuttering: a simple subject experimental design. *Journal of Fluency Disorders* 17, 143–162.

Moore, W.L. and Boberg, E. (1987) Hemispheric processing and stuttering. In: Rustin, L. Purser, H. and Rowley, L. (eds). *Progress in the Treatment of Fluency Disorders*. London: Taylor & Francis.

Mordecai, D.R. (1979) An investigation of the communicative styles of mothers and fathers of stuttering versus non stuttering preschool children. *Dissertation Abstracts International* 40(10), 4759.

Nadirshaw, Z. (1993) Therapeutic practice in multiracial Britain. *Transcultural Psychiatry Society (UK) Bulletin*, Spring 1993.

Nelson-Jones, R. (1988) *Practical Counselling and Helping Skills*. London: Cassell.

Newman, L. and Smit, A. (1989) Some effects of variations in response time latency on speech rate, interruptions and fluency in children's speech. *Journal of Speech and Hearing Research* 32, 635–644.

Pauls, D.L. (1990) A review of the evidence for genetic factors in stuttering. *ASHA Reports* 18, 34–38.

Perksins, W. (1992) *Stuttering Prevented*. Snighlar Publishing Group Inc.

Peters, H.F.M. and Hulstijn, W. (eds) (1987) *Speech Motor Dynamics in Stuttering*. New York: Springer-Verlag.

Peters, T.J. and Guitar B. (1991) *Stuttering: An Integrated Approach to its Nature and Treatment. : Williams and Wilkins.*

Pincus, L. (1976) Death and the Family. London: Faber & Faber.

Prins, D. (1983) Continuity, fragmentation and tension. In: Prins, D. and Ingham, R.J. (eds). *Treatment of Stuttering in Early Childhood: Methods and Issues*. San Diego: College Hill Press.

Rando, T.A. (1984) *Grief, Dying and Death: Clinical Intervention for Caregivers.* Illinois: Research Press

Reisinger, J.J., Frangia, G.W. and Hoffman, E.H. (1976) Toddler management training: generalization and marital status. *Journal of Behaviour Therapy and Experimental Psychiatry* 7, 335–340.

Renfrew, C.E. (1988) *Word Finding Vocabulary Scale*. Oxford: Renfrew.

Riley, G. (1984) *Stuttering Prediction Instrument for Young Children*. Austin, TX: PRO-Ed.

Riley, G. and Riley, J. (1983) Evaluation as a basis for intervention. In: Prins, D. and Ingham, R.J. (eds). *Treatment of Stuttering in Early Childhood: Methods and Issues*. San Diego: College Hill Press.

Riley, G.D. and Riley, J. (1984) A component model for treating stuttering in children. In: Peins, M. (Ed.). *Contemporary Approaches in Stuttering Therapy*. Boston: Little Brown and Co.

Rosenfield, D. and Nudelman, H. (1987) Neuropsychological models of speech dysfluency. In: Rustin, L., Purser, H. and Rowley, D. (eds). *Progress in the Treatment of Fluency Disorder*. London: Taylor & Francis.

Rustin, L. (1987) *Assessment and Therapy Programme for Dysfluent Children*. Windsor: NFER-Nelson.

Rustin, L. and Kuhr, A. (1989) *Social Skills and the Speech Impaired*. London: Whurr.

Rustin, L. and Purser, H. (1991) Child development, families and the problem of stuttering. In: Rustin, L. (Ed.). *Parents, Families and the Stuttering Child*. London: Whurr.

Rustin, L., Fry, J. and Cook, F. (1994) A self-help programme for families of the preschool child for parents who have a first language other than English. *Proceedings International Fluency Conference,* Munich, in press.

Schulman, F.R., Shoemaker, D.J. and Moelis, I. (1962) Laboratory measures of parental behaviour. *Journal of Consulting and Clinical Psychology* 26, 109–224.

Sheehan, J.G. (1975) Conflict theory and avoidance — reduction therapy. In: Eisenson, J. (Ed.). *Stuttering: A Second Symposium*. New York: Harper & Row.

Starkweather, C.W. (1987) *Fluency and Stuttering*. Englewood Cliffs: Prentice Hall.

Starkweather, C.W. and Myers, M. (1979) Duration of subsegments within the intervocalic interval in stutterers and nonstutterers. *Journal of Fluency Disorders* 4, 205–214.

Starkweather, C.W. and Gottwald, S. (1984) Parents' speech and children's fluency. Convention address: American Speech and Hearing Association.

Starkweather, C.W., Gottwald, S.R. (1990). The demands and capacities model II: Clinical Applications. *Journal of Fluency Disorder* 15, 143–158.

Starkweather, C., Gottwald, S. and Halfond, M. (1990) *Stuttering Prevention. A Clinical Method.* Englewood Cliffs, NJ: Prentice Hall.

Stephenson-Opsal, D. and Bernstein-Ratner, N. (1988) Maternal speech rate modification and childhood stuttering. *Journal of Fluency Disorders* 13, 4–50.

Stocker, B. and Usprich, C. (1976) Stuttering in young children and level of demand. *Journal of Fluency Disorders* 1, 116–131.

Till, J.A., Reich, A., Dickey, S. and Sieber, J. (1983) Phonatory and manual reaction times of stuttering and nonstuttering children. *Journal of Speech and Hearing Research* 26, 171–180.

Van Riper, C. (1973) *The Treatment of Stuttering*. Englewood Cliffs, NJ: Prentice Hall.

Van Riper, C. (1971) *The Nature of Stuttering*. Englewood Cliffs, MNJ: Prentice Hall.

Van Riper, C. (1982) *The Nature of Stuttering* (2nd ed). Englewood Cliffs, NJ: Prentice Hall.

Wandsworth and East Merton Health District (1979) *Ethnic Minorities and the Health Service*.

Wall, M. (1977) The location of stuttering in the spontaneous speech of young child stutterers. Ph.D. dissertation. New York: City University of New York.

Wall, M.J. and Myers, F.L. (1984) Clinical Management of Childhood Stuttering. Baltimore, MD: University Park Press.

Wall, M., Starkweather, C. and Cairns, H. (1981) Syntactic influencies on stuttering in young child stutterers. *Journal of Fluency Disorders* 6, 283–298

Weiss, A.L. and Zebrowski, P.M. (1992) Disfluencies in the conversations of young children who stutter: some answers about questions. *Journal of Speech and Hearing Research* 35, 1230–1238.

Wexler, K. and Mysak, E. (1982) Disfluencies in the onset of stuttering. *Journal of Speech and Hearing Research* 27, 154–159.

Wiig, E.H. and Semel, E. (1984) *Language Assessment and Intervention for the Learning Disabled*. Columbus: Charles E. Merrill.

Wood, D. (1986) In: Wood, H., Griffiths, A. and Howarth, C. (eds). *Teaching and Talking with Deaf Children*. London: Wiley.

Wright, L. and Sherrard, C. (1994) Stuttering therapy with British Asian children. Part 1: A survey of service delivery in the UK. Part 2: Speech and language therapists' perceptions of their effectiveness. *European Journal of Disorders of Communication*.

Yairi, E. (1981) Disfluencies of normally speaking two-year-old children. *Journal of Speech and Hearing Research* 24, 490–495.

Yairi, E. (1983) The onset of stuttering in two- to three-year-old children: A preliminary report. *Journal of Speech and Hearing Disorders* 48, 171–178.

Yairi, E. (1993) Epidemiological and other considerations in treatment efficacy resarch with preschool age children who stutter. *Journal of Fluency Disorders* 18, 197–219.

Yairi, E. and Ambrose, N. (1992) A longitudinal study of stuttering in children: a preliminary report. *Journal of Speech and Hearing Research* 35, 755–760.

Yairi, E. and Lewis, B. (1984) Disfluencies at the onset of stuttering. *Journal of Speech and Hearing Research* 27, 154–159.

Yaruss, J.S. and Conture, E.G. (1993) F2 transitions during sound/syllable repetitions of children who stutter and predictions of stuttering chronicity. *Journal of Speech and Hearing Research* 36, 883–896.

Zimmerman, G.N. (1980a) Articulatory dynamics of fluent utterances of stutterers and nonstutterers. *Journal of Speech and Hearing Research* 23, 95–107.

Zimmerman, G.N. (1980b) Stuttering: a disorder of movement. *Journal of Speech and Hearing Research* 23, 122–136.

Index

9 781897 635551